Vaccination

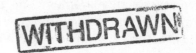

About the authors

Professor emeritus Gordon Ada, AO, DSc, FAA

Gordon Ada spent 20 years at the Walter and Eliza Hall Institute, Melbourne, working first with viruses and then on immunological topics. He then was appointed Head of the Department of Microbiology at the John Curtin School of Medical Research (JCSMR), Australian National University, Canberra working on the immune response to viral infections. During that time, Peter Doherty and Rolf Zinkernagel did the work in the department which later led to the award of the 1996 Nobel Prize in Physiology or Medicine. From 1971 to 1990, he was a member of several committees of WHO involved with vaccine research, development and usage. After retirement, he spent three years at Johns Hopkins University, Baltimore and became Director of a Center for AIDS Research there. He is currently a Visiting Fellow at the JCSMR and has published many articles on vaccines.

David Isaacs MB BChir MD FRACP FRCPCH

David Isaacs is a practising paediatrician, Staff Specialist in Infectious Diseases at the New Children's Hospital, Westmead, Sydney and Clinical Professor at the University of Sydney. He graduated from Cambridge University in 1975 and trained in paediatrics in London and Sydney. He wrote his doctoral thesis on childhood respiratory infections at Northwick Park Hospital, Harrow. He trained in paediatric infectious diseases in Oxford, before moving to Sydney to start a Department of Infectious Diseases at the New Children's Hospital. He was involved with the earliest studies of the new conjugate Hib vaccines in Oxford. He is a member of the Australian Technical Advisory Group on Immunisation (ATAGI), which advises the Minister on immunisations and has been one of the co-authors of the last three *Australian Immunisation Handbooks*. He has written six books and over 150 papers on paediatric infectious diseases, including 50 papers related to immunisations.

This book is a thorough treatise on the global extent of the problem of infectious diseases and the impact of vaccination on them. It addresses, with solid science, the concerns of parents and others in the community who have been vocal against vaccination and informs us of exciting possibilities for the prevention of infectious diseases in the future. Most importantly, from a public health perspective, it contains detailed information for the professional and the parent that is essential for making a fully informed decision about immunisation.

Fiona Stanley AC
Director, Institute for Child Health Research, Western Australia
Professor of Paediatrics, The University of Western Australia

This is the most authoritative and complete book on vaccination written for parents that I have ever seen. Authored by a world authority on vaccination and a leading Australian pediatrician, the book covers virtually every aspect of practical immunology and vaccinology. Physicians as well as parents could profit from reading this book, as the quality of the information is very high. For intelligent parents who have real questions or concerns about vaccination, this is the ideal source.

Stanley A. Plotkin, M.D.
Emeritus Professor of Pediatrics, University of Pennysylvania, Philadelphia

This is an inspired book on one of today's major issues—vaccines. Everything you wanted to know but were afraid to ask—and more! Two world experts, Gordon Ada and David Isaacs, have provided a state of the art exposition on what immunisation is all about—the good and the not so good—no holds barred. It is packed with information, down to earth, immensely readable and, above all, accurate. Anyone who cares about the well-being of family, friends and society should read this wonderful book.

Richard Moxon
Action Research Professor of Paediatrics, University of Oxford

In my work as Chairman of the Advisory Committee overseeing the World Health Organization's global immunisation effort, I see both the extraordinary power of vaccines and the concerns that some parents have about them. What a delight, then, to welcome what is clearly the world's most authoritative, most readable and most balanced book telling the story of vaccines from the very beginning and also peering excitingly into the future. Comprehensive in its scope, richly illustrated, sensibly referenced, it will appeal to students, to concerned parents, to decision makers in the health field and to a wide lay readership. This is not just another book, it is a signal intellectual event deserving to be celebrated. Congratulations to Gordon Ada and David Isaacs, and to Allen & Unwin!

Sir Gustav Nossal
The University of Melbourne

Vaccination

The facts, the fears, the future

Gordon Ada and David Isaacs

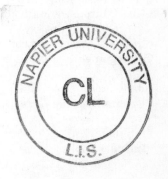

ALLEN & UNWIN

First published in 2000

Allen & Unwin
9 Atchison Street
St Leonards NSW 2065
Australia
Phone: (61 2) 8425 0100
Fax: (61 2) 9906 2218
E-mail: frontdesk@allen-unwin.com.au
Web: http://www.allen-unwin.com.au

National Library of Australia
Cataloguing-in-Publication entry:

Ada, Gordon.
   Vaccination: the facts, the fears, the future.

   Bibliography.
   Includes index.
   ISBN 1 86508 223 6.

   1. Vaccination. 2. Vaccination—Australia. I. Isaacs, David.
   II. Title.

614.470994

Set in 10.5/13 pt Trump Mediaeval by DOCUPRO, Sydney
Printed and bound by McPherson's Printing Group, Maryborough, Vic

10 9 8 7 6 5 4 3 2 1

Contents

Monitoring side effects of vaccines; Cost of vaccine
adverse events; Cost of vaccines; The media; Risks
and benefits

Tables

Figures

Acknowledgements

We wish to thank particularly those people associated with certain institutions and publishing houses who gave permission to us to use diagrams and tables illustrating different parts of this story. These are individually acknowledged where these tables and diagrams are presented, and are listed below. Special thanks are due to Drs Walter Orenstein and Roger Bernier of the Centers for Disease Control and Prevention, Atlanta, GA. USA, for providing information on the incidence of different infectious diseases in the USA this century, and to Dr. Robert Chanock of the National Institutes of Health, Washington, for additional information.

Friends and colleagues read different parts of the work as it progressed and made useful comments—Tony Adams, Robert Blanden, Margaret Burgess, Bill Cowden, Frank Fenner, Kaye Flugelman, Michelle Maxwell, Peter McIntyre, Stanley Plotkin and David Willenborg who read different parts. Phyl and Don Spencer read all the main text. Any mistakes and inaccuracies are however the responsibility of the authors.

We acknowledge the following Organisations for permission to quote from their publications. The World Health Organization, Geneva; Current Biology, London; Office of National Statistics, London; Pediatrics, USA; New Children's Hospital, Westmead; Nature and Society Forum, Canberra; Professor Cedric Mims, UK; Lippincott, Williams and Wilkins, USA.

Preface

Exposure to infectious diseases has always been a major hazard confronting the existence of different forms of life, but especially of humans. This threat to human existence has been clearly documented, ever since the keeping of records. Until very recently, the progress of humankind was determined by the level of survival following epidemics. For example, when first exposed to measles in 1875, more than 40 per cent of the inhabitants of the Pacific island of Fiji died. At the end of World War I, the pandemic (that is, a worldwide epidemic) of 'Spanish' influenza killed more than 20 million people, greater than the number killed by weapons in both world wars combined.

The introduction of the smallpox vaccine in England just over 200 years ago began to change this picture. Within a relatively short time, vaccination to prevent smallpox became compulsory in some European countries such as Bavaria because of the very high level of protection it gave against the disease. But there were many who spoke against the practice. Much later, as smallpox cases became rare in developed countries, complaints began to be raised about the level of unpleasant side-reactions following vaccination. The famed Irish writer, George Bernard Shaw, wrote against the practice, calling it 'a particularly filthy piece of witchcraft'. Some parents refused to have their children vaccinated.

This century, as vaccines became available for other childhood diseases, deaths and illness from these infections became relatively rare. They were so infrequent that students might not see one case of a particular infection during their medical degree course. Thus in the USA in 1921, there were over 200,000 cases of diphtheria. In 1997, there were just five cases!

As the memory fades of many people sick with or dying from these infections and as a new generation who have never seen individuals seriously ill with these infections begins to dominate the child-bearing age group, there have been several developments. Some parents have become so concerned about the side-reactions following vaccination that they resist this practice. Others challenge the basic concept of vaccination. Groups of people who are opposed to vaccination have been formed and increasingly begin to influence parents and parents-to-be with their claims. Some consider that being required to vaccinate their children is an infringement of their rights. Some challenge the scientific basis of vaccination and question whether viruses and bacteria are the cause of some diseases. Some propose that the very low level of some infectious diseases in our society these days is due to the healthier lifestyles which people now lead, and is not due to vaccination against those diseases. There are some who take the point of view that other parents should have their children vaccinated—the more the better—but they do not want their own children to be vaccinated.

In this book, we retrace the history of vaccination and recent information concerning the efficacy of vaccines. We discuss the safety of vaccines in contrast to the risk of serious disease which can result from infection by the naturally occurring viruses or bacteria—information which is generally not widely known and appreciated. The efficacy of a vaccine depends upon the immune response it generates and this is briefly described. Each individual is unique in this respect. Information is slowly accumulating to predict the extent to which a person may be susceptible to or may resist serious disease following a particular infection. In the former case, it is especially important that the person be vaccinated as this will decrease the risk of serious illness or death if that person is subsequently exposed to that infectious virus or bacterium.

The claims concerning the short-term and long-term hazards of vaccination, are compared to the known facts. More frequently now, claims are being made about associations between the occurrence of a disease and a rather earlier vaccination, and these are discussed.

Following a ten-year global vaccination programme, smallpox was shown to be eradicated in the late 1970s and a formal declaration made in 1980. This was a fantastic public health achievement. Based on this success, there is a major effort now to eradicate poliomyelitis with the aim of achieving this by the year 2000. The whole of the Americas has been free of infection by the natural virus since 1991, and progress elsewhere since then has been good. There is considerable hope that it may also be possible to eradicate measles. The collaboration of all countries is necessary to achieve such goals.

There are several challenges for the future. One is to develop effective vaccines against difficult and frequently deadly infectious diseases of global importance, such as HIV/AIDS, malaria and chlamydia. Despite great efforts, this is proving to be quite difficult, but recent advances in our greater ability to manipulate the immune system now offer more hope.

The remarkable success achieved so far in the control of some infectious diseases has led to the hope that the same approach, either as vaccination to prevent the disease, or in the form of immunotherapy (ways of affecting disease by modifying the immune response) of established disease, can be applied to the control of non-communicable diseases. There are now the first clear signs that the immunisation of babies with the hepatitis B vaccine can substantially decrease the later development of and especially the number of deaths due to liver cancer in Taiwan, where the incidence of that cancer is very high. Immunotherapy of some types of cancer, especially melanoma, is looking promising. The first immunotherapeutic treatment of an autoimmune disease, arthritis, is now licensed in the USA. Vaccination also offers an additional method for the control of human fertility, which might be appreciated by different communities. Success has been achieved in one trial in India.

The authors of this book have worked in the area of infectious diseases, and have been involved with aspects of vaccine development or with the practice of vaccination for many years. Both have also had some contact with groups in the community who, as outlined above, are opposed to vaccination. A lot of information about the safety and efficacy of human vaccines against childhood infectious diseases is available in the form of booklets from the Commonwealth Department of Health and Family Services and these are freely available. But we felt that there was a need for information on a broader front which would give a more complete picture about vaccines. Though some of the chapters in the book contain a considerable amount of scientific information, we have tried to present this in such a way that most of those who read the book will grasp the essentials of the immune system and the basis of our arguments.

The book has been divided into two sections. The first section, 'Why vaccinate?' comprises Chapters 1 to 8 inclusive and the second, 'The way ahead', comprises Chapters 9 to 12.

Who would we like to read this book? Anyone who has recently become a parent or plans to become a parent, and has concerns about the practice of vaccination will find it useful. We would especially like those who currently argue against vaccination to come to terms with the scientific, medical and epidemiological evidence presented in the book. But we hope there will also be a broader audience, people of all ages and walks of life, who are interested in reading about what is one of the greatest public health achievements of the twentieth century, understanding how this was achieved and learning about the potential of this technology, vaccination or immunotherapy, in other related areas.

I

Why vaccinate?

1

Infectious diseases of humans

In this chapter, we consider the enormous effect which infectious diseases have had on humans, especially in the past but also in current times. The nature and properties of the common infectious agents which cause disease in humans are described as well as their modes of transmission.

INFECTIONS

From the moment of birth until death we live in an evironment full of infectious agents. Most of these agents cause no ill effects, but a considerable number can cause high levels of sickness and death. But humans and, through humans, their domestic animals, are the only forms of life which have been able to do much about it—and in terms of the period of time of humankind's existence, this has occurred only very recently.

The infectious diseases of people at any one time are a reflection of the living conditions at that time. Until about 12,000 years ago, and for the previous 500,000 years, humans lived in small bands as hunter–gatherers, but had close contact with wild animals. They would have 'shared' infectious diseases with them, such as those caused by rabies (a virus infecting canines) and by salmonella (the bacteria that causes food poisoning in incompletely cooked food) and diseases caused by some mosquito-borne viral infections. With the advent of agriculture and the domestication of some animals, the size of interacting human populations became much larger: big enough to sustain respiratory and sexually transmitted diseases.

As cities with tens of thousands of inhabitants arose, infectious diseases could become rampant. A city such as Rome in the heyday of the Roman Empire had a very high death rate and depended upon continuing immigration of inhabitants from the countryside to maintain its population. Much later, with the provision of clean water, healthy food and sewerage systems, the intestinal infection cholera—a major cause of illness and death—came under control. In Europe this century, cholera has virtually disappeared and so too has leprosy, originally called Hansen's disease, after the Norwegian discoverer of the causative agent (*Mycobacteria leprae*). But cholera epidemics still occur frequently in Third World countries when provision of these services are interrupted, and leprosy occurs in disadvantaged communities such as those of some Indigenous Australians and in several Asian countries. And as the size and proximity of populations increased, respiratory infections such as measles and influenza really took hold and have been with us ever since.

The history of humankind, especially since people began to live in sizable groups, is a series of wars between people and these infectious agents. There have been some remarkable battles which have resulted in the decimation of human populations, but there have always been some survivors to carry on the human race. In his famous book, *Rats, Lice and History*, Hans Zinsser (1935) described the roles of carriers (vectors) of the agents of infectious diseases—the louse and typhus, the flea and the plague and the mosquito and yellow fever. These insects and their deadly cargo had a far greater effect on the destiny of man than did all the machinery used in warfare. In a more recent book, *Guns, Germs and Steel*, Jared Diamond has described the effect of infectious diseases on populations of humans since they began to practise agriculture and domesticate animals some 12,000 years ago in the Middle East and South-West Asia.

Some readers may be familiar with stories about the outbreaks of plague (caused by the bacterium *Yersinia pestis*) which have occurred from time to time. The first of the well documented epidemics began in Constantinople during the

4

sixth century AD, lasted for nearly 50 years and contributed markedly to the downfall of the Roman Empire. At its peak, up to 10,000 people died in a day. Plague reappeared in Europe some centuries later, this time brought by the fleas on rats which hitched a ride in the baggage of travellers on the Silk Road from China and resulted in the greatest plague of all time—the 'Black Death'. About 40 million people, one-quarter of Europe's population at that time, died from the infection.

Viruses have also caused major epidemics. In his recent book, *Viruses, Plagues and History*, the biologist Michael Oldstone has described some of the major outbreaks of diseases caused by viruses, especially in the USA. The Spaniards had a secret weapon when they confronted the Aztecs for the first time in the early 1500s. One of the Spaniards had the smallpox and this caused such a very high and very rapid death rate among the native population, which had had no previous contact with this virus, that there was no chance of effectively resisting even the quite small number of invaders who had survived earlier exposure to the agent. In some areas, up to 50 per cent of the natives died from the infection. Even when present continually in a population, the smallpox virus could cause a high death rate in newly infected people who had not previously been exposed to this virus. At different times after the early settlement of North America by Europeans, exposure to smallpox continued to decimate groups of indigenous peoples.

When measles first reached Fiji last century, up to 40 per cent of the inhabitants died from the infection. A similar pattern was seen when the virus first reached the Faroe Islands, north of Scotland. This pattern of high susceptibility of human populations to an infectious agent is seen when indigenous populations in freshly opened up or exploited habitats are exposed to a 'foreign' infectious agent for the first time.

Australian aborigines suffered greatly from infectious diseases such as leprosy and trachoma introduced by the white settlers, and, in some cases, were deliberately exposed to smallpox. The yellow fever virus caused very high levels of sickness and death in North American cities in the late nineteenth century, and caused a great delay in the building of the Panama Canal.

CURRENT HUMAN INFECTIONS, EPIDEMICS AND
PANDEMICS

Human infections can be classified into two groups—those
which reoccur from time to time according to local conditions,
such as cholera, and those which are new and are hence called
emerging infections. The human immunodeficiency virus (HIV)
is perhaps the best known example of an emerging disease, but
in the second half of the nineteenth century, there also were
outbreaks of infection by the Lassa fever, Ebola and Hanta
viruses. They have caused disease with a very high death rate,
already close to 90 per cent in the case of HIV.

Infections by the influenza virus regularly cause epidemics,
when many people in a region become infected, or a pandemic
when the infection spreads worldwide. The pandemic of 'Spanish flu' which occurred at the end of the First World War caused
more than 20 million deaths, which is greater than the total
number of deaths caused by hostilities during both world wars.
(A recent estimate suggests that the figure might be closer to
100 million.) Infected people could die within 24 hours of
showing clinical signs of infection. The last major pandemic,
the 'Hong Kong' flu, was in 1968. It caused half a million deaths
in that region alone before spreading worldwide. The outbreak
of influenza in humans in Hong Kong (1997) due to infection
by a strain of influenza virus present in the local chickens,
ducks and geese caused a high local death rate in people over
13 years of age and some others had severe complications.
Fortunately, this strain of virus is relatively poorly infectious
for humans (there were fewer than 100 clinical cases, and it
did not spread from person to person), and no further cases of
human infection occurred once the birds in the local markets
were slaughtered. In early 1999, about 100,000 birds in several
large chicken farms near Sydney were slaughtered because of
an outbreak of Newcastle disease, a virus related to influenza
virus. There is a risk that this infection may spread to some
native birds. Fortunately for us, this virus causes at worst only
a very mild eye infection in humans.

Most influenza virus experts believe that another influenza
virus pandemic is certain to occur at some future time. The
actual time is impossible to predict and because of the speed

6

of modern travel, it could spread around the globe at a frightening pace.

THE PROSPECT OF GERM WARFARE

While the prospect of 40–50 million people being infected with HIV by early next century and the possibility of another major influenza pandemic are grim enough, the most frightening current scenario is that posed by biological (germ) warfare, using 'bioweapons' to selectively infect targeted populations. Preston (1998) has described the 'bioweaponeers', especially those from the former USSR who developed a powder containing anthrax bacteria which can travel by air for miles and would likely kill 50 per cent or more of an exposed population. With the breakdown of the USSR and the dispersal of many of the staff involved in this work, there is great concern that some of this material is now held in countries such as Iraq, Syria, Iran and Libya. It has been suggested that a combination of anthrax and the smallpox virus would be very highly effective, because currently, there would be no protection for nearly all of the world's population. Vaccination to prevent smallpox stopped in 1980, and the one vaccine against anthrax for general medical usage is not widely used. It would take a long time to produce enough vaccine of both types to protect large numbers of people.

THE NATURE OF INFECTIOUS AGENTS

There are four main classes of micro-organisms which are capable of infecting vertebrates—viruses, bacteria, parasites and fungi. Some of their properties are now briefly described.

Viruses

Viruses are the simplest and smallest of all biological structures that are able to replicate (reproduce themselves). Outside a living cell, they are inert but inside a susceptible cell, they replicate and produce often hundreds of progeny (offspring) in each cell. Viruses are therefore called obligate intracellular infectious agents, that is, they need cells in which to grow and multiply. Once shed from the infected cell, they have the opportunity to infect more cells in the same or different hosts.

7

They contain either deoxyribonucleic acid (DNA) or ribonucleic acid (RNA) as their genetic material. The RNA or DNA is inside the viral particle and is protected from external damage by a coating of protein molecules. This coat may be made up of a few or many different proteins. Once inside a susceptible cell, the virus 'uncoats', releasing the nucleic acid. Information encoded in the viral nucleic acid is transcribed and/or translated into the different proteins which will become part of the progeny of the virus.

There are substantial differences in size and complexity of virus 'coats'. Frequently, there are a few or many copies of each protein which form the surface of the virus and these pack together symmetrically. Early attempts to make a vaccine to the virus that causes AIDS were unsuccessful because this was not taken into account (discussed in Chapter 10). Some proteins may have carbohydrate (sugar) side chains, and the larger ones may have a lipid (fatty) envelope (covering). They may also contain proteins which have special properties which facilitate or make possible the replication cycle in the infected cell.

Some RNA viruses continually mutate so that new viral proteins are made which differ slightly and may have new 'antigenic specificities'—so that antibody made to the earlier virus might not protect against infection by the mutated virus. This allows the mutated virus to re-infect those who have previously had an infection by an earlier form of the virus. Influenza and the human immunoeficiency virus, HIV, are the main examples of this sequence. Another way of evading the host's immune response is that there may be many serotypes (antigenically different forms) of the same virus in circulation at the same time. One example are the rhinoviruses which are a major cause of the common cold, and this helps to explain why children get so many colds.

The antibiotics used to control bacteria generally do not affect viral growth. That is why effective vaccines are particularly important in minimising sickness and death from viral infections.

Bacteria

Bacteria occupy a position in size between viruses and the cells with a nucleus which are the basic living unit of vertebrates.

Some bacteria replicate inside cells like viruses, but others live and replicate outside cells; the latter therefore have an 'independent' existence. All bacteria contain both DNA *and* RNA. But as is the case with all more complex forms of life (animals and plants), the genetic information that is passed onto their descendants is contained in the DNA. However, unlike the situation in all cells, there is no membrane separating the chromosomal DNA from other cell components (the cytoplasm). The bacterial cell contents are enclosed in a flexible membrane which in turn is enclosed by a more rigid cell wall. Some bacteria, such as salmonella, have long 'tails' called flagella which wave and confer mobility while others have little attachment structures called pili which facilitate adherence to cells. Some bacteria have a capsule or a layer of complex sugars (carbohydrates or polysaccharides) attached to the outside wall; they are called encapsulated bacteria. Some bacteria secrete proteins (called toxins) which are highly toxic to animal cells. These toxins can be made safe (de-toxified) in different ways to form toxoids such as those which form the basis of diphtheria and tetanus vaccines.

As well as having chromosomal DNA, some bacteria contain little circles of DNA called plasmids which may code for resistance to some antibiotics. These can replicate independently of the chromosomal DNA, and can be exchanged between different bacteria. This is how antibiotic resistance can be passed from one bacterium to another.

The discovery of antibiotics enormously enhanced our ability to control most bacterial infections. However, because of their resistance to antibiotics, some bacterial infections can now be very serious and continue to cause brain damage, other long-term consequences and sometimes death. *Mycobacterium tuberculosis*, the bacterium responsible for tuberculosis, is a classic example.

Table 1.1 illustrates the relative differences in size of different viruses, a bacterium and a white blood cell, compared to a tennis ball.

Parasites

'Parasite' is a general term describing infectious agents. Viruses and bacteria are sometimes called microparasites whereas the

Table 1.1   The size of some infectious agents relative to each other and to a tennis ball

Particle	Diameter (nm)*	Relative size (volume)
Poliovirus	27	1
Influenza virus	85	10
Smallpox virus	210–260	290
Small bacterium	750	770
White blood cell	7500	77,000
(lymphocyte)	(10 times the diameter of the bacterium)	
Tennis ball	7,500,000 (10,000 times the diameter of the bacterium)	

*   1 m (metre) = 10^9 nm (nanometres).

protozoa (single-cell animals) and the helminths (worms) are often called macroparasites, or more commonly, just parasites. They come in a great variety of shapes and sizes. Many live outside cells, for example, in blood vessels, but can cause great damage to some cells. Others cause intestinal infections. They vary tremendously in size. At one end of the spectrum, the guinea worm grows to one metre or more in length, and can exit through a hole in the skin of the leg. The malaria parasite is at the other end of the size scale, and in the different phases in its life cycle, the particles vary in size between a large virus or a bacterium.

There is a strong possibility that the guinea worm may be eradicated within a few more years by a rather simple strategy whereas vaccination still offers the best prospect to control malaria (see Chapter 10).

Fungi

The fourth type of infectious agent, the fungi, are extremely widespread and can cause a variety of infections. Such infections are extracellular, that is, they occur within an organism, but not within its constituent cells. Many are restricted to mucosal surfaces (e.g., the cells lining an internal cavity, such as the lung, the intestine or the vagina). Most fungal infections are relatively mild and easily treated with anti-fungal agents. Consequently, vaccine development to control fungal infections has not been a high priority.

A LIST OF COMMON AGENTS CAUSING DISEASE IN HUMANS

Table 1.2 lists the fairly common infectious agents which may infect and cause serious disease in humans. The full Latin names of all bacteria, fungi and parasites are usually written in italics. In contrast, viruses have not been given Latin names. Sometimes, the name of the disease closely follows the name of the agent, e.g. *Mycobacterium tuberculosis* and the disease, tuberculosis, in contrast to *Plasmodium vivax* with the disease, malaria. Sometimes, the name is abbreviated, e.g. *M. tuberculosis*.

Vaccines are available against some of these (indicated by a single star) and rather more are the subject of vaccine development (two stars). For many of the latter however, the work to develop a vaccine is still at the pre-clinical stage (working with experimental models, such as mice or monkeys). For a few others, clinical trials—carrying out tests in humans—have already been performed and registration of the product as a vaccine for medical use may not be far off. Stages in vaccine development—including clinical trials—are described in Chapter 6.

Some viral infections can result either directly or indirectly in certain cancers. The agents involved are indicated in the table and are discussed more fully in Chapter 11. A few viral or bacterial infections can lead to an autoimmune disease, that is, the infection triggers the body's immune system to react against some of the body's own tissues, and so cause disease. Two examples are diabetes and rheumatic fever. Progress in this area is also described in Chapter 11.

Table 1.3 lists the twelve infectious agents, or groups of agents which cause most illness or deaths in the world (1997 estimates). Those groups of agents causing diarrhoea or acute lower respiratory tract infections are really major causes of illness and of death. Of the individual agents, malaria is by far the major cause of sickness. These three, together with tuberculosis and HIV/AIDS are the five major killers. At the current rate of new infections, HIV/AIDS may well top the list of killers within a couple of years. As a single agent, malaria causes most sickness, so it is not surprising that about 40 per cent of the world's population is at risk of catching malaria. At any one

Table 1. 2   Infectious agents causing diseases in humans

Infectious agent	Diseases
Bacteria	
Bacillus anthracis #	Anthrax
Bordetella pertussis *	Whooping cough
Borrelia burgdorferi *	Lyme disease
Chlamydia trachomatis **	Pelvic inflammatory disease in women, (STD)# Blindness (trachoma)
Clostridium botulinuml**	Botulism
Clostridium tetanus *	Tetanus
Corynebacterium diphtheriae *	Diphtheria
Coxiella burnetii *	Severe fever (Q fever) in abattoirs
Escherichia coli **	Diarrhoea
Haemophilus influenzae *	Meningitis, epiglottitis, pneumonia type b (Hib)
Helicobacter pylori **	Gastritis, duodenal ulcer, stomach cancer
Legionella pneumophila **	Legionnaire's disease
Listeria monocytogenes	Meningitis, septicaemia
Mycobacterium leprae **	Leprosy
Mycobacterium tuberculosis *	Tuberculosis
Neisseria gonorrhoeae **	Gonorrhoea (STD)
Neisseria meningitidis **	Meningitis, septicaemia
Pseudomonas aeruginosa **	Nosocomial infections (acquired in hospital)
Tick-borne typhus fever Rickettsia	Typhus. A fever
Salmonella *	Typhoid fever
Shigella **	Dysentery
Staphylococcus aureus **	Impetigo, toxic shock syndrome in women
Streptococcus pneumoniae *	Pneumonia, otitis media (severe fever) meningitis
Streptococcus pyogenes **	Tonsillitis, scarlet fever, rheumatic fever
Treponema pallidum **	Syphilis (STD)
Vibrio cholerae *	Cholera
Yersinia pestis **	Bubonic plague
Viruses	
Adenovirus *	Respiratory disease
Corona virus	Respiratory and gastric disease
Cytomegalovirus **	Mononucleosis (cancer)
Dengue virus **	Dengue fever, dengue shock syndrome
Ebola virus	Haemorrhagic fever
Epstein-Barr virus **	Glandular fever, (infectious mononucleosis), Burkitt's lymphoma (cancer)
Hantaan virus **	Acute lung injury
Hepatitis A*, B*, C, D, E viruses	Liver disease (hepatitis) (cancer)
Herpes simplex virus, type 1 **	Brain infection, mouth lesions
Herpes simplex virus, type 2 **	Genital lesions (STD)

Infectious agent	Diseases
Human herpes virus, type 6	Kaposi's sarcoma (cancer)
Human immunodeficiency viruses, types 1 ** and 2**	Acquired immunodeficiency syndrome (AIDS) (STD)
Human T cell lymphotrophic virus, type 1 **	Cancer of some blood cells
Influenza A*, B* and C	Respiratory disease, influenza
Japanese encephalitis virus*	Brain infection
Lassa fever	Fever, haemorrhage
Measles virus *	Respiratory infection, SSPE#
Mumps virus *	Mumps, meningitis, orchitis (sterility)
Papilloma virus **	Warts, cervical carcinoma (cancer) (STD)
Parvovirus	Respiratory disease, anaemia
Polio virus *	Poliomyelitis, paralysis
Rabies virus *	Rabies
Respiratory Syncytial virus**	Respiratory disease in infants
Rhinovirus	Common cold
Rotavirus *	Diarrhoea in infants
Rubella virus *	German measles, foetal malformations
Smallpox (vaccinia) virus *	Generalised infection (smallpox)
Yellow fever virus *	Jaundice, kidney and liver failure
Varicella zoster virus *	Chickenpox, shingles
Parasites	
African trypanosomes **	Trypanosomiasis, sleeping sickness
Cryptosporidium spp.	Diarrhoea
Entamoeba histolytica	Dysentery
Giardia lamblia	Diarrhoea
Filaria	Elephantiasis
Dracunculiasis	Guinea worm
Leishmania **	Kala azar, tropical sores
Plasmodium **	Malaria
Schistosomes **	Schistosomiasis
Toxoplasma gondii **	Mononucleosis
Trichomonas vaginalis	Vaginal infection (vaginitis) (trichomoniasis)
Fungi	
Aspergillus fumigatis	Pneumonia
Candida albicans	Thrush
Histoplasma	Pneumonia
Pneumocystis carinii	Pneumonia in AIDS patients

*   Licensed vaccine available.
**   Vaccine development in progress.
#   SIDS = sudden infant death syndrome; STD = sexually transmitted diseases; #SSPE = subacute sclerosing panencephalitis, a measles virus induced fatal brain infection.

time, about one-quarter of the world's population (about one and a quarter billion people) are infected with one or more of

Table 1.3   The global health situation—leading causes of serious sickness and of death

Infectious diseases	New cases (incidence)	Deaths
Diarrhoea	4 billion	2.5 millions
Malaria	300–500 millions	1.5—2.7 millions
Acute respiratory infections	395,000 thousands	3.7 millions
Trichomoniasis	170 millions	
Chlamydia	89 millions	
Hepatitis B	67.7 millions	605 thousands
Gonorrhoea	62 millions	
Amoebiasis	48 millions	70 thousands
Whooping cough	45 millions	410 thousands
Measles	31 millions	960 thousands
Tuberculosis	7.25 millions	2.91 millions
HIV/AIDS	5.8 millions	2.3 millions*

*   As AIDS takes up to ten years to develop its full-blown phase and sufferers die at various stages of the illness there wil be many who are diagnosed as HIV-positive who do not yet have AIDS.

Data abstracted from the *World Health Report* (1998), World Health Organization, Geneva.

the parasites that cause malaria, trypanosomiasis, leishmaniasis, schistosomiasis and filariasis. These diseases are characteristically found in tropical countries.

Tuberculosis has recently gained the unenviable title of the main individual killer—nearly 3 million deaths per year. The standard vaccine to prevent tuberculosis, the Bacille-Calmette-Guerin or BCG vaccine is reasonably effective in infants and is a component of the World Health Organization (WHO) Expanded Programme of Immunization (EPI) for children (see Chapter 3). Generally, a tuberculosis infection can be controlled by antibiotics. There are three reasons for the resurgence of sickness and death due to tuberculosis during the last decade: one, failure to keep up with the requirement to constantly and regularly take drugs; two, in developing countries, infection with *Mycobacterium tuberculosis* can be an early death sentence for many individuals with HIV/AIDS; and three, antibiotic-resistant strains have recently become widespread. For example, in the USA and especially in certain areas of New York, there have been outbreaks of this disease in the last decade. It has been estimated that it cost over a billion dollars to bring the recent New York outbreak under control (Coker, 1998).

ANTIBIOTICS AND THE CONTROL OF BACTERIAL INFECTIONS

As well as *M. tuberculosis*, there are continuing problems with antibiotic resistance in the bacteria *H. influenzae, N. gonorrhoeae,* and *N. meningitidis.* (See Table 1.2 for a list of the diseases caused by these bacteria.) This resistance occurs because of one or more mutations in critical proteins. In addition, since 1989, strains of *Salmonella typhi* resistant to multiple antibiotics have continued to spread. The global burden of typhoid fever caused by *S. typhi* is estimated at 30 million cases and 600,000 deaths annually. School age children (5–19 years of age) account for approximately two-thirds of all cases. A WHO committee recommends that either of the two available vaccines for the control of *S. typhi* (see Chapter 3) should be used much more widely as it is known that they are effective in preventing typhoid fever in this age group.

Infection by *Staphylococcus aureus*, the 'golden staph', can be a risk for patients in some hospitals. Resistance to antibiotics by disease-causing bacteria which colonise the gut has become a major problem in Australia and overseas. One antibiotic, vancomycin, has been the major antibiotic to control these infections but recently, vancomycin resistant enterococci (VRE) have been detected in some Australian hospitals.

These examples illustrate the growing concern about the potential for antibiotic-resistant bacteria to create new problems for our already overburdened health system. The development of anti-bacterial vaccines is thus an even more attractive alternative strategy. It is one reason why a special effort is now being made to develop more and better bacterial vaccines (see Chapter 9).

ROUTES OF INFECTION

Infectious agents can infect by several routes, mainly the skin or mucosa—the lining of body cavities and passages such as the intestine. The bites of insects can transmit many infectious agents. In addition to malaria parasites, mosquitoes also transmit other parasites such as filaria, and also a group of viruses—dengue, Japanese and Australian (Murray Valley) encephalitis, as well as yellow fever virus. Rabies is transmitted by the bite of an infected dog or other canine, and some other infections via breaks in the skin. Use was made of this last route towards the end of the Smallpox Eradication Campaign in Africa especially when there was concern that supplies of vaccine were becoming very low. Vaccination with the smallpox vaccine was achieved by pricking the skin several times with a bifurcated needle (like a sewing needle missing the top half of the eye) carrying a drop of the virus solution held by the two little prongs.

However, infection via the mucosa is the major route of most infections. Whereas the skin may have an area of a few square metres, it is estimated that if all the mucosal surfaces of an adult were spread out, they would cover the size of a tennis court! This means that in the body, there is an incredible degree of folding and wrinkling of mucosal surfaces, so that lots of 'niches' are formed where infectious agents—some good, some bad—can 'hide' and live. Thus, there are several different bacteria which live in (colonise) the vagina and some help to protect it from other more dangerous infections.

The main mucosal sites are the intestinal tract (commonly called the gut) with access via the mouth or anus, the lungs (the respiratory tract), the urogenital tract (the vagina and penis), and the eye (ocular route). Infections of the urogenital tracts are called sexually transmitted diseases (STDs) and examples are indicated in Table 1.2. They are very common and are a major cost to society. For example, diagnosis and treatment of pelvic inflammatory disease (PID) of women, in which infection by the bacterium *Chlamydia trachomatis* is a major component, costs several billion dollars a year in the USA. Blindness (trachoma) is caused by infection of the eye by Chlamydia, and hundreds of millions of people worldwide are affected. Other strains of chlamydia can infect the respiratory tract and cause pneumonia.

PATTERNS OF TRANSMISSION OF INFECTIOUS DISEASES

Table 1.4 gives some examples of four major ways in which infections can spread. They include virtually all forms of person-to-person contact, by biting arthropods and infections via contact with animals. Some infections are more readily transmitted than others. Generally, respiratory infections like influenza and measles have a very high transmission rate. Every now and then, there are reports that if a person suffering from influenza boards a plane at the start of a long intercontinental flight, many of the other passengers may be infected by the time the flight ends, especially if it is delayed at one point. Young children are usually faced with significant exposure to infections when they first attend kindergarten. One study reports: 'If you put a small amount of a fluorescent dye onto a finger of a four-year old boy just as he goes into preschool, the dye can be detected at the end of the morning on the books, tables, chairs, doorknobs and on the fingers, mouths and faces of all the other children.' (Mims, 1998) Deep kissing is a perfect way to transfer saliva and so transmit some infections. Sexually transmitted diseases flourish in many societies, in spite of the fact that those caused by bacteria are curable with antibiotics. A recent report (*Lancet*, 1998) stated that the annual incidence of four common sexually transmitted diseases, which are curable with antibiotics, was 1 million in Australasia, 14 million in North America and 16 million in Europe.

This chapter has provided essential background information about the nature of the different infectious agents which cause disease in humans and the way the different infections are transmitted. Earlier this century, before the days of antibiotics and vaccines, it was not unusual for an Australian family with five or six young children living in a house with a safe water supply and with sewerage facilities to lose one or two infants due to infectious diseases. A barefoot youngster cutting a foot by treading on a rusty nail could die from lockjaw—a tetanus infection. Events which were to change that pattern of death by infectious diseases began just over 200 years ago.

Table 1.4 How infections spread

Method of spread		Examples
Person-to-person (direct contact)	Respiratory droplets*	Common cold, influenza, tuberculosis, meningococcal meningitis, measles
	Saliva* or eye discharges	Mumps, glandular fever, certain types of conjunctivitis, including trachoma
	Sexual transmission	Gonorrhoea, HIV, syphilis, genital warts.
	Skin contact (also indirect via dust)	Warts, staphylococcus in hospitals
Person-to-person (indirect contact)	Intestinal infections (eating or drinking contaminated material)	Typhoid, cholera, amoebic dysentery, shigella, virulent types of *E. coli*
	Blood infections, via transfusions, needles	Hepatitis, HIV
Infections from biting arthropods mosquitos, ticks, etc.		Malaria, elephantiasis dengue, yellow fever***
Infections from animals**	via biting arthropods	Lyme disease (ticks on deer), bubonic plague (rat fleas)
	Urine, faeces	Bolivian haemorrhagic fever (mice), Lassa fever, leptospirosis (rats), Giardia.
	Milk	Bovine tuberculosis, brucellosis (cows, goats, pigs)
	Saliva	Rabies (foxes, skunks)
	Inhalation secretions	Psittacosis (parrots, budgies)
	Direct contact with an animal or its hairs, etc.	Q fever, ringworm, anthrax
	Eating vertebrate animal meat (undercooked)	Salmonella, listeria, *E. coli* (e.g. strain 0157)

*   Can also spread via contaminated fingers, handkerchiefs, flies (trachoma).

**   Many of these do not occur in Australia, but exceptions include psittacosis, ringworm, Q fever (in abattoirs), anthrax and salmonella.

***   There are many other viral infections in this category. Murray Valley encephalitis (fever) and Ross River virus (fever, joint pain) occur in Australia.

Modified slightly from Mims (1998). Reproduced with permission from The Nature and Society Forum, Canberra.

2

A short history of vaccines and vaccination

This chapter describes the early vaccination procedures developed to protect humans from a few very serious infections, and how this approach slowly expanded and became a widely accepted procedure.

It was observed in ancient times that those who survived an infectious disease seldom suffered a second, similar sickness. Centuries before the birth of Christ, Thucydides recorded that 'when the plague was raging in Athens, the sick and the dying would have received no nursing at all had it not been for the devotion of those who had already had the plague and recovered from it, since it was known that no-one ever caught it a second time'. As the title of Donald Hopkins' book—*Princes and Peasants: Smallpox in History* (1983)—infers, people in all classes of society were susceptible to infection.

The first exposure to smallpox leaves characteristic pock marks on those who survive. It was observed that repeated exposure to smallpox of surviving individuals resulted in no further sickness or pock marks. Over time, the idea grew that deliberate inoculation with smallpox pustules via a scratch in the skin or inhaled via the nose (variolation) might confer protection without the hazards of natural infection.

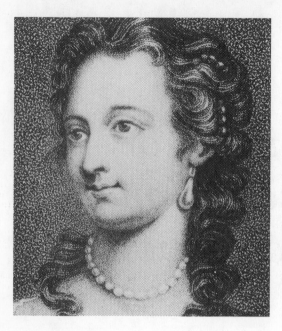

Figure 2.1 Lady Mary Wortley Montagu (1689– 1762) before infection with smallpox (1715). Many high-born ladies, including Lady Montagu, became severely pock- marked after infection. Some wore a mask when appearing in public.
Reproduced with permission from the World Health Organization, Geneva.

THE PRACTICE OF VARIOLATION

This practice originated in China and India and spread westwards. It not only saved lives but became 'commercially' important. In the seventeenth century, the French philosopher Voltaire wrote that to avoid disruption in the trade of young beautiful maidens from Circassia to the seraglios (harems) of the Turkish Sultan and the Persian Sophy during epidemics of smallpox, the Circassians inoculated their female children with 'a pustule taken from the most regular and at the same time, the most favourable sort of smallpox that could be procured'. Lady Mary Wortley Montagu, the wife of the British Ambassador to Constantinople and a notable beauty, became severely pock marked following a smallpox infection (Figure 2.1). Against the advice of the Embassy chaplain who regarded the practice as unchristian, she had her son inoculated, and he was protected against further exposure to smallpox in this way. She took the news and the evidence back to London (her daughter was inoculated there), and in due course, the practice spread in England and thence to the Americas. Figure 2.2 indicates the much stronger reaction to variolation compared to the cowpox inoculation which was introduced later.

Figure 2.2. **The Gold-Kirtland drawings of the extent of reaction 11 days after inoculation of the arm by variolation or by vaccination. Variolation induced a much more severe reaction.**

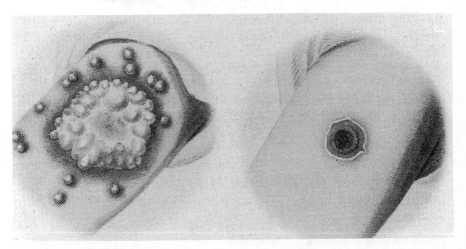

Reproduced with permission from the World Health Organization, Geneva.

By current-day standards, the practice of variolation (named after the variola virus which causes smallpox) was a rather desperate undertaking as the fatality rate was 0.5–2 per cent, but this must be compared with 20–30 per cent after natural smallpox infection. Ten per cent of all deaths in London during the seventeenth and eighteenth centuries were due to smallpox. In the nineteenth century, the British historian, Thomas Macaulay, described the ravages of the disease: 'tormenting with constant fears all whom it had not yet stricken, leaving on those whose lives it spared the hideous traces of its power, turning the babe into a changeling at which the mother shuddered, and making the eyes and cheeks of the betrothed maiden objects of horror to the lover'. No wonder Macaulay called smallpox 'the most terrible of all the ministers of death.' And in his autobiography, the eminent American, Benjamin Franklin lamented:

> In 1736, I lost one of my sons, (Francis Folger) a fine boy of 4 years old by the smallpox. I long regretted bitterly and still regret that I had not given it to him by inoculation. This I mention for the sake of parents, who omit the operation on the supposition that they should never forgive themselves if

the child died under it: my example shows the regret may be the same either way, and that therefore, the safer should be chosen.

Variolation did cause many concerns and in the early nineteenth century in England, following the adoption of the much safer procedure of using cowpox (see below), it was made a crime to carry out variolation on human beings.

EDWARD JENNER AND THE BEGINNING OF THE END FOR SMALLPOX

In the second half of the eighteenth century, it became clear that milkmaids in some European countries including England, frequently escaped smallpox disease, as illustrated in the following poem:

> Where are you going to, my pretty maid
> I'm going a milking, sir, she said
> May I go with you, my pretty maid
> You're kindly welcome, sir, she said
> What is your father, my pretty maid
> My father's a farmer, sir, she said
> What is your fortune, my pretty maid
> My face is my fortune, sir, she said.

It came to be realised that the milkmaids were protected from smallpox infection because of an earlier mild infection acquired from cows. A farmer in England, Benjamin Betsy, who worked with cows, inoculated his wife and children with material obtained from the pocks on cows. They were protected from smallpox for about 15 years. But it was Edward Jenner who in 1796 carried out the definitive test. He inoculated a young boy, James Phipps, first with cowpox and later deliberately with smallpox to see if he was protected. The boy was completely protected and this finding ushered in the current era of immunisation. The practice spread rapidly and the protection afforded against smallpox was so dramatic that some European countries made inoculation compulsory early within the next century. Napoleon Bonaparte was so impressed by the effectiveness of this procedure that he declared that he could not refuse Dr Jenner any request!

Once smallpox began to disappear from developed countries, concern was increasingly expressed about the level of side effects or adverse reactions following vaccination. This concern persisted right up to the successful completion of the Smallpox Eradication Programme in the late 1970s. The worry about side reactions became a general feature of vaccination programmes once the incidence of people suffering from the original infection had fallen to low levels.

THE MANY CONTRIBUTIONS OF LOUIS PASTEUR

The second great advance in developing vaccination as a valid and safe public health procedure was made by the great French scientist, Louis Pasteur. He established that infections were caused by small micro-organisms or microbes—the germ theory of disease. (It was previously believed by many that infections began spontaneously out of the air.) The museum in the Pasteur Institute in Paris contains examples of the techniques used by Pasteur in his work. He discovered (initially by accident) the means of changing the properties of microbes so that their potential for causing disease (their virulence) was greatly reduced. This process is now called *attenuation* and has been a major technique for developing vaccines especially against viruses. Pasteur realised that in some respects, cowpox could be regarded as an attenuated form of smallpox. In honour of Jenner, he coined the terms vaccine and vaccination (*vacca* is Latin for 'a cow') to apply to immunisation procedures used to protect against any infectious disease. He developed vaccines against chicken cholera and anthrax for protecting birds and animals. The anthrax vaccine was tested on cows, sheep and a goat at a public demonstration at Pouilly-le-Fort. Vaccinated and non-vaccinated animals were given a lethal dose of anthrax. To the astonishment and delight of the public, all the vaccinated animals survived whereas all the others died. This result announced to the world that a new era in vaccination had been achieved.

Rabies was a common disease of dogs in Europe at that time and anyone bitten by a rabid dog was very likely to die. Pasteur was able to attenuate the infectious microbe (later identified as a virus) by sequentially growing (passaging) it many times in rabbit brains. In 1885 when confronted by a boy, Joseph Meister,

23

Figure 2.3   **An English engraving by James Gillray, 1802, reflects the scepticism with which vaccination was received initially in some quarters. It shows the outpatient department of a hospital. On the left, those to be vaccinated are being given a purgative; on the right, those already vaccinated, their faces contorted with pain, are turning into cows, the source of the vaccine.**

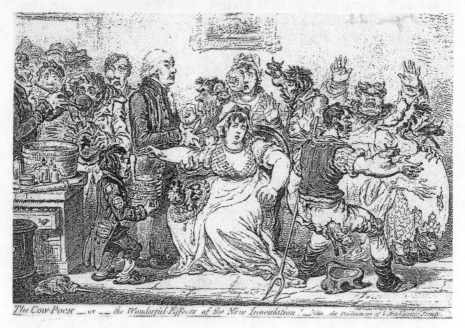

The Cow-Pock _ or _ the Wonderful Effects of the New Inoculation ! _ Vide .the Publications of ŷ Antivaccine Society.

Source: Fenner, F. et al. (1988). *Smallpox and its Eradication.* World Health Organization, Geneva.

who had been bitten by a rabid dog and was considered certain to die, Pasteur made the courageous decision to inoculate him with his attenuated preparation. Joseph's life was saved. There was immediately a public outcry that the process of vaccination with a live infectious microbe had been applied to a human. Some of Pasteur's closest scientific friends were appalled and temporarily deserted him, despite the fact that subsequently many human lives were saved by his procedure. It was alleged that some patients died from the vaccination, but it would have been very difficult to prove that this was the case, because all the patients had previously been bitten by a rabid dog. (Immunisation against rabies is one case where a vaccine can be given with a protective effect *after* the infection has occurred because rabies has a long incubation period.)

Figure 2.4   An anti-vaccination poster from Britain, 1906.

THINK

of the unparalleled ab-
surdity of deliberately infecting the organism of a
healthy person in this day
of **SANITARY SCIENCE**
AND ASEPTIC SURGERY
with the **POISONOUS**
matter obtained from a
sore on
A DISEASED CALF!

JOIN THE   J. W. HODGES, M.D.

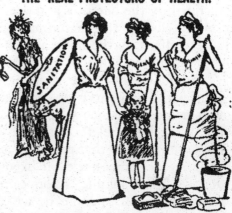

THE REAL PROTECTORS OF HEALTH.

NATIONAL ANTI=VACCINATION LEAGUE,

50, PARLIAMENT STREET, WESTMINSTER, S.W.

Nevertheless, vaccination was accepted more readily on the Continent than in Britain where there was fierce opposition well into the twentieth century. Figure 2.3 reflects the scepticism with which vaccination against smallpox was viewed in some quarters. This was partly due to lack of proper control of vaccine quality, and the realisation that a single inoculation did not give lasting protection, as Jenner had claimed. Many groups believed that the decrease in smallpox cases was due to improved sanitation and living conditions (Figure 2.4).

Once it was shown that killed (inactivated) bacteria could also protect from other diseases, the next three vaccines which were developed were all inactivated bacterial preparations, namely the different bacteria causing typhoid and cholera (1896) and the plague (1897).

ANTIGENS AND ANTIBODIES

By this time, some researchers were growing bacteria in a liquid medium in the test tube. In the case of the diphtheria bacteria, it was found that if the bacteria were then removed (by filtration), injection of the liquid itself (the filtrate) could still protect against the disease normally caused by those bacteria. The filtrate was shown to contain a toxic protein (toxin) secreted by the bacteria and was recognised as specific antigen associated with the bacterium. An antigen is a substance which is recognised by the body as being foreign, and hence different to its own components.

At about the same time, it was found that the blood of people who had survived an infection, or had been successfully vaccinated, contained soluble factors which would cause clumping of (agglutinate) the bacteria. Most importantly, transfusion of the serum from that person to another could protect the latter, at least for some weeks, if exposed to the agent causing that disease. These soluble factors came to be called *antibodies*, and the part of the microbe to which they bound was called an *antigen*. We now know that a small virus, such as polio, might contain five or six different antigens, a large virus (smallpox) about one hundred and a bacterium, several hundreds of different antigens. Studies early in the twentieth century showed that antibodies had exquisite specificity. An antibody might no longer react with an antigen if the latter had only been slightly modified. A later most surprising finding was that the body could make antibodies to artificial antigens—structures which were entirely novel and different from any naturally occurring products. (This process is described in Chapter 4).

OTHER VACCINES DEVELOPED BEFORE WORLD WAR II

Prior to 1940, two live attenuated vaccines were made—BCG (1927) described in Chapter 1, and yellow fever (1935). It is difficult these days to appreciate the tremendous amount of work involved in developing these vaccines. Isolated from a patient in 1927, the yellow fever virus was passaged in sequence as follows: 53 times in monkeys, followed by 58 times in baby mouse cells, and finally 160 times in embryo chicken cells, making sure no brain cells were present in the latter cell mixture. The virus was also passaged several times in mosquitoes. (This number of passages was required to derive a strain of virus which had lost its capacity to induce disease and to grow in brain cells and hence would not infect the human brain.) It was a heroic achievement and the yellow fever vaccine remains to this day a very effective and safe one.

The first pertussis (whooping cough) and rickettsia inactivated bacterial vaccines and the influenza virus vaccines were developed and licensed during this period. The influenza virus was grown in fertile (containing embryos) hens' eggs, a technique which is still used. Finally, in the 1920s the two toxoid vaccines to protect against diphtheria and tetanus were developed by treating the toxins with chemicals such as formalin to detoxify them while retaining their ability to induce a strong protective antibody response. Both vaccines have been remarkably effective. For example, as previously mentioned, there were over 200,000 cases of diphtheria in the USA in 1921. In 1997, there were only five cases of this frightening disease.

POST WORLD WAR II VACCINE DEVELOPMENT

World War II marked a turning point in many areas important for vaccine development. Most of the vaccines used in vaccination programmes today were developed after 1945. The ability of John Enders and his colleagues in the USA in the early 1950s to grow the polio viruses in cultures of identical cells made it possible to grow many other viruses and, in turn, to develop vaccines leading to the control of these diseases. A list of these vaccines is given in the next chapter. Making attenuated strains of the different viruses has remained a remarkably effective way to develop effective viral vaccines, even to this day. Four vaccines based on inactivated (as opposed to infectious, attenuated) viral preparations were also developed. A contributing factor to this success with vaccine development was the great advance in our knowledge of the body's immune system and the new techniques of molecular biology.

With the exception of anti-viral drugs against herpes viruses, there are no *widely* used drugs available for the control of other viral infections. New generation drugs—'designer drugs'—to control infections such as HIV and influenza are only now becoming available. But the commercial production of antibiotics has generally been remarkably successful in controlling bacterial infections, and this has lessened the incentive to make bacterial vaccines.

The development of live attenuated or inactivated bacterial vaccines has been relatively difficult, and until recently, making what are called subunit preparations has been more successful. In this method, only part of a bacteria or a virus is used as the basis of the vaccine and the different approaches are described in Chapter 3.

Of particular interest has been the development of hepatitis B vaccines. Hepatitis B virus (HBV) is a human pathogen (disease-producing organism) which can cause chronic infection and may result in cirrhosis or liver cancer in children but the highest incidence is in middle age. About 300 million people worldwide are infected, and they live mainly in Southeast Asia. People may be infected for life, and a pregnant infected woman can pass on the infection to her child at birth. The virus does not grow in tissue culture (cells grown outside the body which can support the production of intracellular viruses or bacteria). The blood of infected people contains both infectious virus particles and the surface antigen of the virus particle. The latter proved suitable as the basis of a vaccine, but in isolating it from the blood, very great care had to be taken to inactivate any live virus which might contaminate the product. Because of this ever present danger, a new approach was taken. The newer techniques of molecular biology made it possible to introduce the DNA coding for the hepatitis B viral surface antigen, called HBsAg, into yeast cells. As the yeast grows and the cells divide, each cell will also produce HBsAg which can be separated and purified. The pure HBsAg is the basis of the vaccine used mainly in developed countries. In this vaccine, there is no possible chance of contamination with live virus, and any slight contamination with yeast proteins should cause no harm. It is the first genetically engineered vaccine and has proved to be successful, relatively inexpensive and very safe. A second genetically engineered vaccine, this time to control Lyme disease—the symptoms of which include arthritis, skin lesions, neurological and cardiac damage—has recently been licensed for use in the USA.

EARLY INDICATIONS OF THE SUCCESS OF SOME CURRENT VACCINES

The Centers for Disease Control and Prevention (CDC) in Atlanta, Georgia, USA, have kept records for many years on the incidence of different infectious diseases in that country. Two examples are now quoted which show the extent of disease reduction shortly after the introduction of the two relevant vaccines. The first measles vaccine was licensed in the USA in 1963. Before then, the annual number of cases of measles from 1912 onwards was *always* greater than 100,000 with a peak number of 894,134 cases during a major epidemic in 1941 (described in Chapter 5). Four years after the introduction of the vaccine, the number of cases had dropped to 62,705, and decreased steadily from thereon as the vaccine became more widely used. The triple combination vaccine, measles-mumps-rubella (MMR), was introduced in the 1970s. By 1981, the number of measles cases had dropped to 3,124.

In 1952, three years before the first polio vaccine—the Salk vaccine—became available, there was an epidemic of poliomyelitis with 21,269 cases of virus-induced paralysis (total cases of illness: 57,879). By 1957, the number of cases had dropped to 5,485 and by 1960, to 3,190 cases.

THE GLORIOUS AND DARKER SIDES OF VACCINE DEVELOPMENT

The tremendous achievement of vaccines, especially of childhood vaccines, in saving human lives is described in Chapter 5. This has only been achieved by the very hard work of devoted biomedical scientists and their colleagues. Since the initiation of Nobel Prizes in 1896, no less than 13 have been given for scientific work of direct relevance either to actual vaccine development or understanding how vaccines work (see Table 2.1). The special significance of some of these scientific advances will be discussed in Chapters 4 and 5.

But along the way, there have been darker episodes. Handling some infectious agents can be very dangerous and many devoted workers have accidentally been infected and paid the ultimate price for their efforts. There have also been fatal accidents among those receiving the vaccines. These have sometimes been due to imperfectly prepared and tested products. The list includes polio, rabies, smallpox and yellow fever viruses, and BCG (tuberculosis) and diphtheria bacterial preparations. For example, the first batch of inactivated polio

Table 2.1   A list of Nobel Prize Laureates in Medicine or Physiology for findings related to vaccine development.

Year	Recipient(s)	Topic
1901	E. A. von Behring (G)*	Serum therapy against diphtheria
1905	R. Koch (G)	Studies on tuberculosis
1908	P. Ehrlich (G) I. Metnikov (R)	Properties of cells involved in immune reactions
1919	J. Bordet (B)	Antibody and complement can kill bacteria
1930	K. Landsteiner (Au)	The exquisite specificity of antibodies
1951	M. Theiler (SA)	Isolation of yellow fever virus
1954	J. F. Enders (US) T. H. Weller (US) F. C. Robbins (US)	Growing polio virus in tissue culture (isolated cells) (This opened the way to make many other viral vaccines)
1960	F. M. Burnet (Austr) P. B. Medawar (GB)	The discovery that immunological tolerance is acquired before birth
1972	G. M. Edelman (US) R. R. Porter (GB)	The demonstration that antibodies have light and heavy polypeptide chains, and domains with different functions
1980	B. Benacerraf (US) J. Dausset (F) G. D. Snell (US)	The establishment of inbred lines of guinea pigs and of mice. This made possible the demonstration that the immune response is genetically controlled
1984	N. K. Jerne (D) G. J. F Kohler (G) C. Milstein (GB)	Development and control of the immune system; The ability to clone B cells which make antibodies of a single specificity
1987	S. Tonegawa (US)	How genes re-assort to generate antibody molecules
1996	P. C. Doherty (Austr) R. M. Zinkernagel (Sw)	How T cells recognise virus-infected cells, resulting in their destruction

*   G = Germany; R = Russia; B = Belgium; Au = Austria; SA = South Africa; US = USA; Austr = Australia; GB = Great Britain; F = France; D = Denmark; Sw = Switzerland.

vaccine prepared by one manufacturer contained some live virus and this resulted in some deaths in the vaccinated group. On another occasion, batches of BCG were improperly labelled, with disastrous results. Fortunately, the list is not very long, but one productive outcome was the establishment of supervisory authorities by governments to regulate the standards of purity and potency of biological products, including vaccines. In Australia, this is the Therapeutic Goods Administration (TGA); in the USA, it is the Food and Drug Administration (FDA) and both of these bodies have very high standards.

But the complete safety of a vaccine only becomes certain when it has been given to very large numbers of people. One example shows that a global authority, the World Health Organization, has high standards. In many developing countries, the measles virus is endemic, that is, always present in the community so there are frequent outbreaks. Babies receive anti-measles antibody from their mother before birth (across the placenta), and this passively acquired immunity may be enhanced by breastfeeding. The measles vaccine is not effective in the presence of this antibody, so the vaccine is not given until nine months of age, which is an average time for the antibody level to decrease to a low enough value for the vaccine to be effective. But for some babies, this low value is reached between six and nine months, so they are susceptible to natural infection during this period. It is estimated that hundreds of thousands of babies in developing countries still die from measles because of this. So the question was—can a slightly stronger vaccine be used which will be effective if given at six months? Such a vaccine was made, and in the early trials in some developing countries, the vaccine induced a good immune response in six-month-old infants and appeared to be safe. But when used on a rather larger scale, a few deaths occurred, restricted to baby girls living in very poor districts in impoverished countries. An investigation showed that the children probably did not die of measles but from other, later infections. However, a doubt remained—so it was decided by WHO that the new vaccine should not be used at all. The ability to save the lives of so many children each year depends upon developing a different type of measles vaccine. It would need to be effective in the presence of specific antibody so that it could be given soon after birth. As measles is one of the human infectious diseases that we may be able to eradicate from the world, solving this problem became a priority. How this is now being achieved in some developing countries is described in Chapter 7.

In developed countries, infants are usually not exposed to measles in the first year of life, and they receive the measles vaccine by itself or in the combination MMR vaccine at 12–15 months of age.

The next chapter describes the types and properties of the different vaccines currently in use, the schedule for their use in Australia and elsewhere, and a list of infectious agents for which vaccine development is well advanced.

3

Current vaccines and vaccination procedures

This chapter describes the properties of current vaccines and those close to registration for medical use. The Australian and some international schedules for childhood vaccination are also given. The use of this technology for prophylaxis (vaccination prior to infection occurring) versus therapy (after infection has occurred) is discussed, as well as the usefulness of passively acquired immunity (transfer of specific serum to give short-term protection against a particular disease agent).

VIRAL VACCINES

There are three types of viral vaccines—live (infectious), attenuated preparations; inactivated (non-infectious) whole virus preparations; and subunit (only part of the virus) preparations. Table 3.1 is a list of those registered for human use, presented under the above headings together with an indication of their efficacy and the usual routes of transmission versus vaccination. Of the attenuated preparations, most have been available for many years. Because of the global eradication of smallpox (see Chapter 7), vaccinia (smallpox vaccine) is available in very limited amounts and kept mainly for an emergency. The adenovirus vaccine is used only in the US Armed Forces, but is included here because although it is given orally, it protects against respiratory infection. Others such as the varicella

Table 3.1   Current viral vaccines

Type	Efficacy	Route of administration	
		Infection	Vaccination
Live attenuated virus			
Smallpox (vaccinia)*	High	Mucosal	Intra-dermal
Yellow fever**	Very high	Mosquito	Injection
Polio (OPV)	Very high	Oral	Oral
Measles	Very high	Respiratory	Injection
Mumps	Very high	Respiratory	Injection
German measles (rubella)	Very high	Respiratory	Injection
Rota	High	Oral	Oral
Chickenpox (varicella)*	High	Respiratory	Injection
Adeno*	High	Respiratory	Oral
Inactivated whole virus			
Influenza*	Variable, but generally high	Respiratory	Injection
Cholera**	Moderate, short duration	Oral	Injection
Polio (IPV)	High	Oral	Injection
Japanese encephalitis**	Moderate to high	Mosquito	Injection
Rabies*	High	Skin (bite)	Injection
Hepatitis A*	Moderate	Faecal, oral	Injection
Subunit			
Hepatitis B (HBsAg)**	High	Mucosal, skin	Injection
Influenza*	Variable, but generally high	Respiratory	Injection
Combination			
Measles, mumps, rubella (MMR)	High	—	Injection

OPV = oral polio vaccine; IPV = inactivated polio vaccine.
Unstarred vaccines are part of the childhood immunisation schedule.
*   Vaccines for specific use;
**   Vaccines to be taken before travel to countries where these infections occur more regularly, for example, China.

(chickenpox) and rotavirus vaccines are recent additions. All these vaccines were first licensed in the USA. Currently, an Australian rotavirus candidate vaccine is in clinical trials in Melbourne. This is a very appropriate development as this virus was first discovered by scientists at the University of Melbourne.

There are five inactivated viral vaccines. Whereas the oral polio vaccine (OPV) is given orally, and is used worldwide, especially in the programme to eradicate poliomyelitis (described in Chapter 7), the inactivated polio vaccine (IPV) is used in some developed (mainly European) countries. The inactivated polio vaccine is more expensive than the oral polio vaccine, but its use avoids the very rare occurrence of paralysis following the administration of oral polio vaccine. The influenza vaccine is mainly recommended for the elderly. The current rabies vaccine is made from virus grown in tissue culture. Hepatitis A, like hepatitis B, also causes liver disease, although the two viruses are very different. There are a number of other viruses causing liver damage, and one, hepatitis C, is now the subject of much study.

The yeast-derived hepatitis B vaccine was described earlier (Chapter 2), but for reasons of cost, preparations made from infected blood are still made and used in some developing countries. The subunit influenza vaccine contains only the two 'surface' antigens of the virus, and following injection, gives a milder reaction than the whole virus vaccine, especially in children.

Several features are characteristic of the diseases controlled by all vaccines. Firstly, with the exception of hepatitis B, the other infections are 'acute', that is, the infections usually don't persist. Death or recovery within a week or so follows a natural infection. Secondly, with one exception, the antigens in the viruses remain 'constant'—they don't vary in their specificity—so that there is only one strain or, in the case of polio, three strains. However, the influenza virus can show great variation (Chapter 1), and that is why a new vaccine, closely matching the currently circulating strains, is made each year.

From the manufacturers' point of view, subunit vaccines are attractive because of their potentially very high level of safety. Despite the higher possibility of adverse reactions (see Chapter 6), live attenuated preparations usually have a very high efficacy. The viral vaccines in late stage development are in this category—a remarkable testimony to the efficacy and safety of the current attenuated viral vaccines. The list includes new influenza, hepatitis A and Japanese encephalitis virus preparations, as well as cytomegalo, dengue and parainfluenza virus preparations.

BACTERIAL VACCINES

Table 3.2 lists the current bacterial vaccines and although each type of vaccine is represented, the numbers in each category are quite different compared to those in the table of viral vaccines. Until fairly recently, BCG was the only live, attenuated bacterial vaccine, but since its introduction, the Ty21a typhoid vaccine has proved to be very effective in protecting against *S. typhi*, the cause of typhoid. Other mutant strains of this bacteria and an attenuated *V. cholerae* preparation may soon be licensed. The *B. pertussis* whooping cough vaccine is generally quite effective but complaints about side reactions and adverse effects (Chapter 6) led to the development of subunit (acellular) vaccines, initially in Japan but later in the USA and Europe. A new inactivated *V. cholerae* preparation administered with a highly effective adjuvant (a substance which enhances the immune response to the vaccine) will likely shortly replace the older cholera vaccine.

The tetanus and diphtheria bacteria cause sickness and death because of the toxic proteins (toxins) they secrete. The ability to 'detoxify' these toxins was a major advance, because it made possible the development of highly effective vaccines. As part of the triple vaccine combination DPT, they are administered with the adjuvant, alum (aluminium salts), the only one approved for general medical usage.

In the case of encapsulated bacteria, i.e. those with a sugar (polysaccharide) coating, it has been possible to make vaccines using all or part of the polysaccharide as the main bacterial antigen. While these vaccines are effective in adults, young children give a poor response (for reasons which will be discussed in Chapter 4). This has been overcome by attaching (conjugating) the sugar part to a protein antigen, acting as a 'carrier'. Young children respond much better to these conjugates, as evidenced by the great success of the *Haemophilus influenzae* type b (Hib) vaccine when introduced into Australia a few years ago (Chapter 5).

Fortunately, bacteria don't show the type of rapid mutation (antigenic drift) seen in some RNA viruses, such as influenza and HIV. But they can exist as different serotypes, each displaying different antigenic specificities. Thus, there are about 100

Table 3.2 Current bacterial vaccines

Type	Efficacy	Route of administration	
		Infection	Vaccination
Live, attenuated bacteria			
BCG, a vaccine to control tuberculosis*	Variable	Respiratory	Injection
Typhoid (*S. typhi*, Ty21a)**	High	Oral	Oral
Inactivated, whole bacteria			
Whooping cough (*B. pertussis*)	High (generally)	Respiratory	Injection
Cholera (*V. cholerae*)**	Low	Oral	Oral
Plague (*Y. pestis*)**	?	Fleas	Injection
Toxoid			
Tetanus (*Cl. tetani*)	Very high	Skin break	Injection
Diphtheria (*C. diphtheriae*)	Very high	Respiratory	Injection
Q fever (C. burnetii)*	High	Respiratory	Injection
Subunit			
Whooping cough (acellular)	High	Respiratory	Injection
Typhoid (Vi polysaccharide)**	High	Respiratory	Injection
Lyme disease (recombinant OspA) (*Borrelia burgdorferi*)*	High	Ticks	Injection
Polysaccharide/protein conjugate			
Pneumococcal (*S. pneumoniae*)*	High	Respiratory	Injection
Meningococcal, Hib (*H. influenzae*, type b)	Very high	Respiratory	Injection
Combination			
Diphtheria, tetanus, pertussis, (whole cell, DTPw)	Very high		Injection
Diphtheria, tetanus, acellular pertussis (DTPa)	Very high		Injection

Unstarred vaccines are those in the childhood vaccination schedule.
*   Vaccines used for other requirements, excluding travel;
**   Vaccines to be taken before travel to countries where these infections can occur more regularly.

different *S. pneumoniae* strains, and the current vaccine contains 23 of these different strains—those which are most common in the USA and cause most disease.

Tables 3.1 and 3.2 show several similarities. Although most microbes infect via a mucosal surface, frequently the respiratory route, most vaccines are given by injection. There are several reasons for this. Administering the correct dose of vaccine is more certain, and often a longer lasting immune response occurs after one or two doses. Sometimes, administering a vaccine by a mucosal route induces only a short-lived response. However, mothers and children dislike injections so increasing research is being carried out on combining vaccines—combinations like the triple antigens MMR or DPT are already widely used—so as to minimise the number of injections required. But there is more research now on improved methods for immunising via mucosal surfaces, especially the respiratory and oral routes (Chapter 9).

In other respects, the vaccines described in Tables 3.1 and 3.2 fall into three groups—childhood vaccines, those for more specific use (for example, influenza for the elderly), and those which may be administered before travel to countries where the particular diseases occur more regularly, as indicated in the footnotes to the tables.

One Australian-developed vaccine has proved to be quite successful. The bacterium *Coxiella burnetii* causes Q fever, a debilitating disease that is particularly prevalent in abattoir workers. A South Australian group led by Professor Barry Marmion made an inactivated whole organism vaccine. It causes a severe reaction in those who have already been infected by the natural microbe. However, by not vaccinating workers who have been shown by a blood test to have been previously exposed to this organism, others not previously exposed have been successfully vaccinated using this vaccine.

A very large amount of work has been carried out towards developing vaccines against some parasites, especially malaria. Some candidates have undergone clinical trials, but none has yet successfully passed final clinical trials. So, it will be some time before such vaccines are generally available for travellers to or residents of malarious countries (see Chapter 10).

COMBINATION VACCINES

As mentioned above, many people, but especially young children and their parents, dislike a needle injection. So there is much work in progress to see if different vaccines can be combined and so limit the number of injections. Another advantage would be less visits to the doctor or health centre. To make such combinations is quite tedious work as it must be established that adding an extra preparation to an existing combination does not interfere with the efficacy of any component. Some combinations are available in different countries now. For example, both hepatitis B (Hep B) and *H. influenzae* type b (Hib) have been combined. The most ambitious project has been to combine hepatitis B, Hib and diphtheria, tetanus and whole cell pertussis (DTPw) (whooping cough), to form the pentavalent (i.e. containing five components) vaccine DTPw-HepB-Hib. It is expected that a similar combination, but replacing whole pertussis with acellular (subunit) pertussis—DTPa-HepB-Hib—would soon become available. When some of the newer approaches to vaccine design become established, making vaccine combinations should be less of a problem.

IMMUNISATION SCHEDULES FOR CHILDHOOD VACCINATION

The WHO Smallpox Global Eradication Programme began in 1966 and by the early 1970s was beginning to show signs of real success in African countries. By then, it had become very clear to the WHO teams that the sickness and death rates of infants from common childhood infectious diseases in these countries was very much higher than in a country like the USA, where a childhood vaccination programme had been in place for some time. As a result, the WHO decided to initiate a special programme to immunise infants in developing countries with six vaccines—tetanus, diphtheria, whooping cough, measles, polio and BCG (tuberculosis). The infant vaccination coverage in these countries at that time was less than 5 per cent! The programme—called the WHO Expanded Programme of Immunization (WHO/EPI) began in 1974. UNICEF joined the programme and, by purchasing very large quantities of vaccine at one time was able to provide them at an incredibly low cost—less than US$1 for all vaccines per person! The hepatitis B virus vaccine was later added at an extra cost. The recommended immunisation schedule is given in Table 3.3.

By 1990, an estimated 80 per cent of children in developing countries reaching their first birthday had been vaccinated with DPT, oral polio vaccine, measles and where it was approved, with BCG. This had involved over 500 million contacts with children. By 1992, it was estimated that some 3 million infant deaths had been averted, as well as some 400,000 cases of poliomyelitis. Considering the difficulties involved, this is a

Table 3.3   WHO/EPI recommended schedules for the immunisation of infants

Contact	Age of child	Vaccines
1.	At birth	BCG, OPV, and HBV^A *
2.	6 weeks	DTP, OPV, and HBV^{AB}
3.	10 weeks	DTP, OPV, and HBV^B
4.	14 weeks	DTP and OPV
5.	9 months	Measles and HBV^{AB}

BCG = for the control of tuberculosis; DTP = diphtheria-tetanus-pertussis vaccine; OPV = oral poliovirus vaccine; WHO/EPI = World Health Organization Expanded Programme for Immunization.

* The hepatitis B virus (HBV) vaccine schedule is flexible. Schedule A (HBV^A) is recommended for populations for whom there is a significant risk of perinatal transmission. Schedule B (HBV^B) is recommended for populations for whom this risk is minimal or immunisation at birth is not possible. A third dose of HBV vaccine may be given at 9 months if necessary.

remarkable achievement. Although the goal is now 90 per cent coverage, this has so far been difficult to achieve.

WHO has a number of other special programmes on vaccine development and usage. Most of the funds for these programmes come from developed countries. In addition, a group called The Children's Vaccine Initiative (CVI) was formed in 1990. Based in Geneva and working in association with WHO, The United Nations Development Programme, the World Bank and the Rockefeller Foundation, they outlined plans to reduce the incidence of different infectious diseases for children in developing countries to specific levels by the year 2000. They identified certain problems requiring special attention in the 1990–2000 decade and the goals they hoped to achieve. These included:

- poliomyelitis—global eradication by the year 2000;
- neonatal tetanus (a major cause of death during child-birth in developing countries)—a major reduction by immunisation of over 90 per cent of women of child-bearing age;
- measles—reduction of deaths by 95 per cent and of cases of disease by 95 per cent;
- diarrhoea—reduction of 50 per cent in children younger than five years of age;
- acute respiratory infections—reductions by one-third of deaths in children less than five years of age.

Table 3.4   Australian standard vaccination schedule (NHMRC, 2000)

Age	Diseases/agents	Vaccine
Birth	Hepatitis B	Hepatitis B vaccine
2 months	Diphtheria, tetanus, pertussis	DTPa
	hepatitis B, *H. influenzae*, type b	HBV, Hib (PRP-OMP)
	poliomyelitis	OPV
4 months	Diphtheria, tetanus, pertussis	DTPa
	hepatitis B, *H. influenzae*,	HBV, Hib (PRP-OMP)*, OPV
	poliomyelitis	
6 months	Diphtheria, tetanus, pertussis	DTPa
	hepatitis B**, poliomyelitis	HBV, OPV
12 months	Measles, mumps, rubella	MMR
	H. influenzae	Hib (PRP-OMP)
18 months	Diphtheria, tetanus, pertussis	DTPa
	poliomyelitis	OPV
4–5 years	Diphtheria, tetanus, pertussis	DTPa
	poliomyelitis, measles-	OPV, MMR
	mumps-rubella	
15–19 years	Diphtheria, tetanus, pertussis	DTPa
	poliomyelitis	OPV

*   Hib (PRP-OMP) indicates the particular vaccine used.
**   hepatitis B at 6 or 12 months

The major targets in the last two categories are rotavirus infections causing diarrhoea, and respiratory syncytial viral (RSV) infections. The first rotavirus vaccine was licensed in the USA in 1998. (The CVI programme was disbanded in early 1999 when WHO took over many of the activities.)

The Australian schedule for childhood vaccination is presented in Table 3.4 and in more detail on pp. 207–9 (Appendix 2). There are substantial differences between WHO/EPI and the Australian schedules, a very important one being that in the latter, a second dose of measles vaccine (as MMR) is given. This is now recognised as being critical. Infection with the natural measles virus usually results in lifetime protection from a second infection. The vaccine protects about 95 per cent of children, but this means that each year there is a build-up of susceptible children. If measles is introduced into schools, an outbreak can occur among those immunised children who did not respond well enough to the first shot of vaccine. Such outbreaks can be predicted mathematically, and can be averted by giving a second dose of measles vaccine to school age children. This was done successfully in the United Kingdom

Table 3.5   Recommended Australian adult–elderly immunisation schedule

Age (Time)	Vaccine
Every 10 years	DT (adult)
Post-partum for non-immune women	Rubella or MMR
Over 50 years (Aborigines)	Pneumococcal (every 5 years) influenza (yearly)
Over 65 years (all)	Pneumococcal (every 5 years) influenza (yearly)

Data taken from the *Australian Immunisation Handbook*. (6th edition) (1997). NHMRC, Canberra.

in 1997. To avoid the flow-on of an epidemic of measles which occurred in early 1998 in New Zealand, the Australian government, to its credit, initiated a mass measles vaccination programme of school age children who were given a second dose of MMR (measles-mumps-rubella) in late 1998. A similar epidemic in Australian children was thus prevented. In future years, a second dose of MMR will be routinely administered at 4–5 years in order to reduce the number of susceptibles and avoid outbreaks. As will be seen in Chapters 5 and 7, this approach has had a remarkable effect on the incidence of measles in some other countries.

The most recent revision to the Australian Standard Immunisation Schedule recommended by the Australian Technical Advisory Group on Immunisation is attached as Appendix 2.

The other major differences between developed and developing countries are the BCG vaccine which is routine in developing countries but only used for a few high risk children in developed countries, and Hib vaccines which cannot yet be afforded by developing countries.

Table 3.5 shows the schedule for vaccines to be administered to adults and the elderly.

Maternal versus neonatal (foetal) vaccination

A baby is usually protected from some infectious diseases for about nine months after birth due to transfer of maternal antibodies to the foetus from the mother via the placenta, and by breastfeeding after birth. This will be the case in countries where many diseases such as measles are endemic (continually present), or when the mother has earlier been successfully vaccinated. This protection can be enhanced by re-vaccinating the mother during pregnancy. This approach has been quite successful in the veterinary industry in protecting offspring from several serious infections.

In some developing countries, there is an enhanced death rate especially of the baby at childbirth due to tetanus infections if the umbilical cord is severed under non-sterile conditions. Vaccination of pregnant women against tetanus in order to reduce this death toll has become a major goal of the WHO. Polysaccharide-based vaccines such as *H. influenzae* type b (Hib) and the pneumococcal vaccines (Table 3.2) have been administered to pregnant women without any adverse effects. This has resulted in increased levels of specific antibodies in the infant. This approach is being seriously considered for general use in those countries where the pneumococcal bacteria are a leading cause of death of infants. It is unlikely that attenuated viral or bacterial vaccines will be used for this purpose, as they are potentially slightly more risky for pregnant women.

PASSIVELY ACQUIRED IMMUNITY IN ADULTS

The presence of specific antibody is the only way to prevent a particular infection (discussed in Chapter 4). Serum obtained from people who have had the infection or been vaccinated (immune serum) or the antibody isolated from that serum (antibody fraction) is regularly used to give short-term (2–3 weeks) protection from a given infection. One major use is the protection of travellers going on a short trip to a country where the disease is common. Hepatitis B infection is endemic in many Southeast Asian countries, and if there is a risk of accidental exposure to the hepatitis B virus an injection of antiserum beforehand should give protection.

In those countries, a baby can be exposed to hepatitis B virus at birth if the mother is infected. Even though the vaccine is given at birth, it takes a week or so for the subsequent immune response to be effective. Transfer of immune serum in addition to vaccination at birth gives protection during this period, and so increases the efficacy of the vaccine. In contrast to the measles vaccine (a live attenuated virus), the hepatitis B vaccine is still effective when antibodies are present.

Several other sera or antibody fractions are available. They include normal immunoglobulin, anti-chickenpox, anti-rabies, anti-tetanus and anti-cytomegalovirus preparations. The passive transfer of specific immune serum is an important technology for protecting and saving lives, especially if it is too late to vaccinate.

In view of the seriousness of an HIV infection, attempts have been made to see if vaccinating an infected person (a process called immunotherapy) with a potential anti-HIV vaccine would either cure the infection or ameliorate the disease process. So far, such attempts have been unsuccessful, for reasons which will be discussed in Chapter 10. However, there is about a 25 per cent chance (or a higher chance in some developing countries) that a child born to an HIV-infected mother would be exposed to the virus during birth and become infected. If twins were born, the risk is higher for the first-born child. In developed countries, this risk has now been greatly reduced by dosing the expectant mother with an anti-HIV drug called AZT during pregnancy. For developing countries especially, there are large programmes underway to see if transfusion of high levels of anti-HIV antibodies to the mother before birth will also protect the baby from infection during birth.

As will be discussed in the next chapter, antibody is usually not very effective in curing an already established intracellular infection. However, certain types of cells, called cytotoxic T lymphocytes or 'killer' T cells which are formed during an infection and sometimes after vaccination, can often kill already infected cells before new virus or bacteria are formed. There are many examples of this effect in model systems with laboratory animals, but now, there are some human examples where transfer of such cells has proved to be beneficial. For example, most of us are infected with cytomegalovirus (CMV), but specific killer T cells control but do not completely clear the infection. If a person is to receive a transplant, (of foreign bone marrow cells for example), the immune system of the recipient is deliberately suppressed so that the foreign cells are then not rejected. However, this now allows the cytomegalovirus to replicate and disease to occur. To combat this problem, in one series of cases, some other cells (lymphocytes) from the donor person were removed shortly before transplantation took place. These cells were activated in tissue culture to become killer cells and then transferred to the recipient of the transplant. Having now full anti-cytomegalovirus activity, these transferred cells were able to kill CMV-infected cells and so keep the virus in check, so that CMV-induced disease did not occur.

The efficacy of a vaccine depends almost entirely on the immune response that is generated in the vaccinated person. The nature and magnitude of the response will vary from person to person as the immune response to foreign material such as a vaccine is genetically controlled and we all have different collections of genes. This has important implications for vaccine design and efficacy and is discussed in the next two chapters.

4

How vaccines work
The immune response
to infectious agents
and vaccines

Opponents of vaccination sometimes claim that immune responses to infections or to vaccines are not important. As part of their argument, they point to the fact that some children who have been vaccinated against a particular infectious disease may still become sick when later exposed to the natural infection. This observation is quite correct, but there is a scientific reason for such occurrences. In order to understand more about vaccination, we first need to understand how the immune system works—which is what this chapter outlines. It is a complicated but fascinating story. Based on this understanding, Chapter 5 presents data confirming the overall efficacy of vaccines and explains why some people respond less well to some infections and to some vaccines. Readers should try to understand the essentials of this system in order to appreciate the rationale of the newer approaches to vaccine development (Chapter 9).

In order to survive, all organisms must have means of combating infectious agents. The more complex the organism, the greater the variety of the mechanisms which have evolved to protect the organism. In the case of humans, the process of vaccination depends upon taking advantage mainly of one of our two major types of defence systems.

Because the mammalian immune system is quite complex, this chapter is divided into two main parts. Part 1 provides a summary of the main points. Part 2 spells out the information in more detail (but still a simplified version) for those who would like to have a greater understanding of how the system works. It describes the work of particular scientists, many Australian, and some of whom have been awarded the Nobel Prize in recognition of their contribution to our knowledge and understanding.

Part 1—A summary of the main features of the adaptive immune system

1 There are two systems—the 'innate' system which can come into operation very quickly; and the adaptive system which takes time to be activated. Only the latter shows great specificity in its response and develops memory (like the brain). Vaccination activates and depends on the adaptive system.

2 In order to combat an infectious invader, what the body needed was an immune system which would mainly do two things: one, produce substances which would *specifically* recognise the invader as being foreign, bind to it and so prevent infection. Antibodies, produced by *B* lymphocytes, do this job. Two, if some of the infectious invader did infect host cells, a special cell was needed which, by surveying the outside of the host cell, would recognise that it was infected and hence 'dangerous', and kill it. CD8 *T* lymphocytes do this and are called *c*ytotoxic *T* *l*ymphocytes (*CTLs*) or killer T cells.

3 B lymphocytes, coming directly from the *b*one marrow, and *T* lymphocytes coming from the *t*hymus, do their work in lymph nodes. While in the thymus, most T lymphocytes capable of recognising *self* proteins/antigens (i.e. of host origin) are destroyed. By the time B and T cells reach the lymph node, they are mature, can recognise foreign antigens and be activated by contact with them.

4 Once activated, B cells make and secrete antibody. Each B cell makes antibody of a single antigen-binding specificity. They may bind antigen directly through antibody receptors

of that specificity on their surface, and produce an antibody called IgM (Ig is short for immunoglobulin). It is the first type of antibody produced during an infection. More often, the B cells react with an activated T lymphocyte; this 'helps' the B cell to make other types of antibodies, such as IgG, IgE or IgA. They have different roles to play in the body.

5   Antigen-presenting cells (APCs, such as dendritic cells—see the glossary) take up much of an invading foreign antigen— virus, bacterium or vaccine, and carry it to the nearest lymph node where it meets with T lymphocytes.

6   If the antigen is non-infectious (for example, a dead virus particle), the APC will break it down to smaller units, called peptides (a string of amino acids). A peptide may combine with a protein in the cell called a class II major histocompatibility (MHC) protein. The peptide:MHC complex, after being formed inside the cell, is presented at the surface of the APC. This complex is recognised by a receptor on a T lymphocyte with a CD4 marker. Once activated, type 2 CD4 T lymphocytes specifically interact with and help B lymphocytes make different antibodies, as described above. They do this by secreting a particular pattern of hormone-like proteins, called cytokines. In contrast, once activated, type 1 CD4 T lymphocytes secrete quite a different pattern of cytokines. Importantly, they help another T lymphocyte which possesses a different marker, CD8, to become mature.

7   If the invader, say a virus, is not dead, but alive and infectious, it can infect the APC. Some of a newly synthesised viral protein is broken down to peptides and some may combine with class I MHC proteins, and this complex is then expressed at the cell surface. If a mature CD8 T lymphocyte (CTL) recognises this peptide/MHC complex on the APC (or on almost any infected cell) as being an altered and not a self pattern, it kills the cell, generally before new infectious progeny is formed and released by the infected cell.

8   Thus, the role of the MHC on the cell surface is to alert the host's immune system to a possible change in the body's cells, from being self-like (normal) to being foreign or 'altered self' (abnormal) and hence a potential danger to the host. However, MHC molecules are extremely variable and

each individual has only a small selection of a total huge number, so that antigenic peptides may or may not bind to those MHC molecules available in the cell. Thus the ability to respond to any antigen is genetically determined.

9 This system has memory; if re-exposed to the same infectious agent, the body remembers and makes a more rapid and greater immune response.

10 Following an infection, a CTL response occurs and usually controls and clears an infection before specific antibody is made in quantity. But because antibodies and not CTLs have the potential to *prevent* an infection, vaccines to date have been designed mainly to induce high levels of specific antibody. However, in order to cope with other more difficult infectious disease challenges, scientists are looking at alternative strategies. (Chapter 10).

Part 2 A more complete explanation of how the immune system responds to infections and to vaccines

There are two protection systems; one is called the 'innate' or inborn system, and the second is called the adaptive system. It was originally thought that these were two completely distinct systems, but it is now realised that they are quite closely integrated. Both are rather complicated but in this chapter, we explain the basic aspects of each.

THE INNATE SYSTEM

All multicellular organisms, including plants, have evolved mechanisms to protect themselves against an infection. In the simpler systems such as invertebrates, the defence system involves the production of soluble factors by host cells which are more harmful to the invader than to the host. In higher species, such as the vertebrates, the innate system is more complex, consisting of different cell types, and a range of factors produced by these cells. These factors are given different names. One group of factors is collectively called cytokines, meaning different proteins produced and secreted by cells. Other smaller-sized factors are called chemokines. Some of these different factors affect the behaviour of other cells, for example, by making them more resistant to infection by viruses or bacteria or influencing their patterns of movement. Other factors are directly harmful to the invading viruses or bacteria. Different cells have different roles in this system. One cell type, the macrophage, is very effective at swallowing and destroying infectious agents as well as damaged or dead cells—it is a scavenger, and this process is called phagocytosis (literally 'eating cells'). But sometimes, the macrophage is tricked, and the infectious agent (e.g. the bacterium causing tuberculosis or the virus causing AIDS (HIV), can live and replicate in this cell. Another cell type, the natural killer (NK) cell, can under certain circumstances recognise infected cells and destroy them, but the conditions for this are rather restricted. Furthermore, this cell may not distinguish between cells infected by different viruses or bacteria.

The most important point about the innate system is that components can come into operation within minutes or hours of an infection occurring. Some bacteria can grow and divide every 20 minutes so that the population may double in size every 20 minutes. We depend upon the innate system to keep the infection from becoming really serious because the adaptive sytem takes some time (days, weeks) to become effective, and finally clear or better control the infection. As an example, one such mechanism depends upon the cell type called the neutrophil. These cells are made in the bone marrow, at the rate of *10 billion* each day. They circulate around the body and secrete factors which can kill bacteria but each cell has a lifespan of only about 10 hours. But each day, the body has to expend enough energy to produce this large number of cells in part on the off-chance that a bacterial infection may occur at any time!

THE ADAPTIVE OR SPECIFIC IMMUNE SYSTEM

Early in Chapter 2, a quotation from Thucydides described the occurrence of the plague in ancient Athens, well before the birth of Christ. The essential point in this statement was that those who got this disease and recovered from it never suffered the same disease again. This clearly demonstrates the first of the two critical characteristics of the adaptive immune system—namely, long-term memory. The body learns from the first infection—somehow it remembers. The Thucydides quotation infers the second critical aspect—even though a person might never have another attack of the plague, they could still suffer from other diseases because the memory about plague is specific. Thus, *memory* and *specificity* are the two hallmarks of the adaptive system. The next section describes the cells involved.

CELLS WHICH HAVE IMPORTANT ROLES IN THE ADAPTIVE IMMUNE RESPONSE

Mainly two types of cells are involved. The first cell type is called the lymphocyte, so called because it is by far the major cell type found in the lymph vessels which deliver the lymphocytes from the tissues to the lymph nodes. In the lymph nodes and in the spleen, the lymphocytes are exposed to antigens, are activated and differentiate into 'effector' cells. For example, the so-called B lymphocytes differentiate to become plasma cells whose sole job is to make and secrete antibodies with particular specificities. Similarly, the final stage of differentiation of T lymphocytes is to have effector activities such as cytotoxicity (ability to recognise and then kill infected cells), or to 'help' B cells make different antibodies. Once they have fully differentiated, the effector cells leave the lymph nodes via other lymph vessels and travel to different parts of the body via the blood.

The second type of cell is called an antigen-presenting cell (APC). Two very important ones are also part of the innate system, the macrophage (which we have already met) and the dendritic cell (DC). The latter used to be called a 'veiled' cell because its plasma membrane has many folds and so has a very large surface area. The macrophage breaks down particles such as viruses and bacteria into smaller units such as proteins, which after excretion may bind directly to the appropriate B lymphocyte. The dendritic cell is especially good at breaking them down into smaller units, called peptides (strings of amino acids).

Mainly B lymphocytes

B lymphocytes are so-called because they travel directly to the node from the *bone* marrow. In contrast, T lymphocytes migrate from the bone marrow to the *t*hymus (a small organ near the top of the chest, above the heart) which they leave in due course to travel to the lymph node. They are called T lymphocytes—T for thymus. (Frequently, these lymphocytes are also often simply called T and B cells). The bone marrow and thymus are called *primary* lymphoid organs, because this is where the lymphocytes are made and undergo the process of 'education' to become competent. Consequently, the B lymphocytes which leave the bone marrow and the T lymphocytes which leave the thymus are fully competent to do their job; in their different ways, they can recognise and respond to foreign antigen. The phrase 'immunocompetent but naive' is often used to describe these cells. 'Immunocompetent' means they are now capable of recognising antigen; 'naive' infers that they have not yet interacted with specific antigen. Similarly, an adolescent might be called sexually competent but naive, if he or she has not yet experienced sexual intercourse.

The spleen and lymph nodes are called secondary lymphoid organs, because that is where the lymphocytes meet with antigen and become effector cells (that is, no longer naive).

Altogether, it is thought that about a thousand billion different antigenic patterns can be recognised by B lymphocytes—an extraordinarily large repertoire! Initially, there were different concepts about lymphocytes making antibodies. In 1957, Macfarlane Burnet in Melbourne made the then heretical proposal that an individual B lymphocyte made antibody of only a single antigenic specificity. This implied that *all* antibody molecules which could be produced by a particular lymphocyte would have the same structure (sequence of amino acids). It would therefore only recognise an antigen with the correct complementary structure (the lock and key analogy). This was completely against the dogma of the time. The background to this proposal is outlined in Table 4.1.

It took ten years before the extra laboratory-based findings became available which showed that this concept was correct! The same pattern of specificity applies to the antigen-recognising receptor on T lymphocytes (a single specificity/cell).

The proof of this concept with B lymphocytes had two important implications. First, because of the tremendously wide variety of antigen-recognising patterns in any population of

Table 4.1   The development of the Clonal Selection Theory of Antibody Formation (Burnet, 1957)

1901. Paul Ehrlich (Nobel Laureate, 1906)
Some cells had 'side chains' which would bind an antigen. When that happened, the cells would make many more of the side chains and secrete them into the blood. (These side-chains are now called antibodies.)

1930s. Karl Landsteiner (Nobel Laureate, 1930)
Antibodies were highly specific, and they could be made against entirely synthetic antigens which never existed naturally. This seemed to show that Ehrlich's idea was wrong; why should the body have the ability to make an antibody against an antigen that before now had never existed? To accommodate Landsteiner's finding, others proposed that the antibody molecule was very flexible and that once an antigen entered the cell, the antibody molecule would 'mould itself' around the antigen (acting as a template), and so gain that particular specificity. This was called the Template Hypothesis. Originally, there seemed to be some experimental evidence to support this concept but it was later shown that these experiments were faulty.

1955. Niels Jerne (Nobel Laureate, 1984)
Antibody molecules of many different specificities occurred naturally without the specific antigen being present. When an antigen:antibody complex was formed, it could be phagocytosed by and stimulate that cell to make more of that antibody.

1956. Dave Talmage, USA
Antigen *selected* a cell with antibody receptors which matched the specificity of the antigen. The cell then replicated and made more of that receptor (antibody)—like Ehrlich's proposal. Talmage noted that antibody made by a B cell tumour had a very constant amino acid sequence.

1957. Macfarlane Burnet (Nobel Laureate, 1960)
From when it was first proposed, Burnet always thought the Template Hypothesis was wrong. It could not explain the existence of immunological tolerance and also his early finding (1928) that when a second dose of antigen was administered, there was a very rapid and large (logarithmic) increase in the production of antibodies (the secondary response). He then proposed an entirely new concept—the Clonal Selection Theory—which suggested that an individual B lymphocyte had antibody receptors of a single specificity. When antigen matching that specificity bound to that cell, it induced a clonal expansion in cell numbers, resulting in strong antibody production. Exposure to a second dose of antigen induced a further great expansion in those cell numbers, thus explaining the great increase in antibody production in a secondary response. The production of antibodies against self molecules (the breaking of self tolerance) was 'forbidden'.

Burnet regarded this theory as his greatest scientific contribution. It is now regarded as the central paradigm of immunology. Immunologists continue to regard it as absolutely fundamental to our understanding of how the immune system works.

B and T cells, some of the patterns recognised by some B or T cells will be the same as or very similar to patterns of host components. This means that a strong immune response could be made against host proteins (called an autoimmune response), resulting in very serious illness and probably death. This was a particularly serious potential problem for T lymphocytes. Fortunately, it came to be recognised that in the few days spent in the thymus, most T cells which recognise the patterns of host proteins die. Thus, of every 100 precursor T lymphocytes which travel from the bone marrow to the thymus, about 95 die there and only about five leave as immunocompetent cells. This process of death of cells recognising self antigens is called immunological tolerance (tolerance to self) which is discussed later. The process is not perfect as reactions against many self antigens can still occur, e.g., autoimmune reactions such as diabetes in humans, but the great majority of vertebrates survive and reproduce despite the occurrence of autoimmune diseases.

Burnet predicted that because the newborn's immune system would need to be able to cope with infectious agents almost immediately after birth, this process of tolerance to self antigens would need to be learnt before birth. Peter Medawar and colleagues carried out the following experiment to see whether Burnet's prediction was correct. If skin from adult strain A mice was transplanted onto adult strain B mice (A and B were quite different strains of mice), the cells in the transplant were recognised as foreign by strain B mice, and the transplant was rejected. If bone marrow cells from strain A mice were injected into newborn strain B mice (i.e., at birth), a subsequent transplant of A strain skin onto these treated B mice when they became adults was not rejected. This experiment is illustrated in Figure 4.1. In other words, contact at birth with antigens on the foreign cells resulted in lasting tolerance to them. Thus, Burnet's concept was shown to be right, and he and Medawar shared the 1960 Nobel Prize for this concept and its proof (as noted back in Table 2.1).

The second implication of this concept relates to the structure of antibodies. Antibodies are proteins and the central dogma of molecular biology states that each protein is coded for by a specific DNA sequence. However, if antibodies of a thousand billion specificities were each coded for separately by DNA, an unusually high proportion of the DNA in a cell would be required just to code for those molecules. This would be quite an impractical situation.

Figure 4.1   Self tolerance is learnt before birth

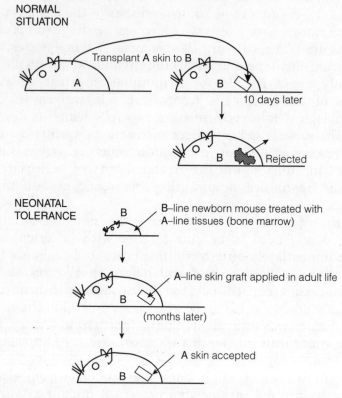

Peter Medawar and colleagues Leslie Brent and Rupert Billingham conducted these seminal experiments in the 1940s and 1950s. The experiments demonstrate that the introduction of foreign cells from bone marrow during early neonatal development can induce a state of acquired immunological tolerance. The system is tricked into treating the foreign tissue as self.

Figure reproduced with permission from E.J. Steele, R.A. Lindley and R.V. Blanden (1998). *Lamarck's Signature*, Allen & Unwin, Sydney.

In the 1960s, the structure of the commonest antibody, immunoglobulin G (IgG), was shown to be two long or heavy (H) peptide chains and two shorter or light (L) peptide chains. Each chain has one region where there is great amino acid variability; this is the part, the antigen-binding site, which recognises antigenic patterns. The rest of each chain has a far more constant amino acid sequence, some parts of which are recognised by receptors on cells so that the antibody/antigen complex would bind to those cells. Rodney Porter and Gerry Edelman shared the 1972 Nobel Prize for these findings about antibody structure (Table 2.1). Susumu Tonegawa was awarded the 1988 Nobel Prize (Table 2.1) for showing that in humans and in mice, smaller pieces of DNA coding for different regions of L and H chains could combine in different ways to give the great variation in antibody specificities, with a great saving in the total amount of DNA required for coding these molecules. These findings are outlined in Figure 4.2.

On leaving the bone marrow, B lymphocytes migrate around the body via the blood and lymph but spend time in the secondary lymphoid organs—the spleen and the different lymph nodes. This is where they generally meet with foreign antigen and with T lymphocytes—and become effector cells.

INTERACTION OF ANTIGEN WITH B LYMPHOCYTES

When activated after binding antigen, the task of B lymphocytes is to make and secrete antibodies. The commonest antibody is immunoglobulin G (IgG) whose basic structure is shown in Figure 4.2 (the term immunoglobulin is synonymous with antibody). Before meeting with antigen, the cell expresses on its surface a larger antibody molecule, IgM, which has ten antigen-binding sites. (It also expresses another antibody, IgD, but little is known about its role.) The B cell may bind the foreign antigen directly via IgM, and this can result in production and secretion of more IgM antibodies of that specificity. More frequently, the B lymphocyte will interact with a T lymphocyte which has already met with and 'processed' the same antigen (see below). As a result, the B lymphocyte now is further activated, differentiates and expresses and secretes one of the other antibody molecules, IgG, IgA or IgE. IgA has four antigen-binding sites. On its passage to a mucosal surface, for example that lining the gut, it is converted to secretory IgA (s.IgA) which is secreted into the gut. There, it can meet with and can bind directly to a virus such as poliovirus, and so prevent the virus from infecting a host cell. Fortunately, s.IgA is very resistant to damage by enzymes which are digesting protein foods in the gut. Other antibody molecules, IgG and IgE are secreted by activated lymphocytes 'inside' the body (Table 4.2).

Figure 4.3 summarises the major events which occur within

Figure 4.2   Structure and formation of the IgG antibody molecule
(i) Structure

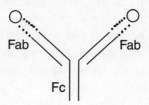

<table>
</table>

Heavy chain (H), constant region ——
Heavy chain (H), variable region ....
Light chain (L), constant region ——
Light chain (L), variable region . . . .

The two top arms of the molecule are called the Fab (fragment, antigen-binding), and the bottom segment, Fc (fragment which could be *crystallised*, because it had a constant amino acid sequence). The Fc fragment contains amino acid sequences, which are recognised by molecules on a cell surface (receptors), so allowing an antigen:antibody complex to bind specifically to that cell, be engulfed (phagocytosed) and degraded. Different segments of the L and H chain variable regions come together to form the antigen combining sites, O.

(ii) Formation of an immunoglobulin heavy chain

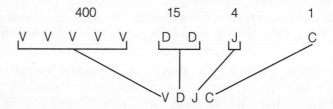

Parts of the H chain are encoded in different and separated pieces of DNA in one chromosome. One of each of the 400 different V (variable) DNA sequences, the 15 different D (diversity) DNA sequences and the 4 different J (joining) DNA sequences randomly come together and link with the DNA coding for the C (constant) chain to form a linear DNA molecule which codes for a linear H chain (VDJC). About 24,000 different combinations are thus possible. A similar situation occurs with the L chain. There is thus the opportunity for any individual L and H chain to come together and to form a complete antibody molecule. This explains how antibody molecules expressing about a billion (24,000 x 24,000) different antigen-binding specificities can be produced. As the C regions of different classes of antibodies vary only slightly and account for 75 per cent of the H chain and 50 per cent of the L chain, much less total DNA is required compared to the amount if all antibody molecules were separately coded for.

Susumu Tonegawa received the 1988 Nobel Prize for elucidating this mechanism.

a lymph node where the lymphocytes interact with the foreign antigen following an infection. It should give the reader some idea of the incredible intricacy and efficiency of the events leading to the formation of effector T and B cells.

Table 4.2   The types, properties and roles of different antibody molecules

Type	Number of antigen-combining sites (ACSs)	Roles
IgM	10	First antibody made; individual ACSs* have only moderate affinity, but with 10 sites, it can bind very well. IgM and complement can lyse many bacteria.
IgG	2	Major antibody formed after infection or vaccination; can become highly specific (affinity maturation); there are several sub-types.
s.IgA#	4	Major means for preventing infection, e.g., by polio virus, at a mucosal surface.
IgE	2	Activates some cells involved in the control of parasite infections; can cause severe inflammation.

*   antigen combining sites of antibodies
#   In the tissues, this antibody occurs as IgA, but on passage to a mucosal surface, it complexes with a molecule (s) which allows it to be secreted through cells lining the mucosa.

Figure 4.3   Events in a lymph node during infection

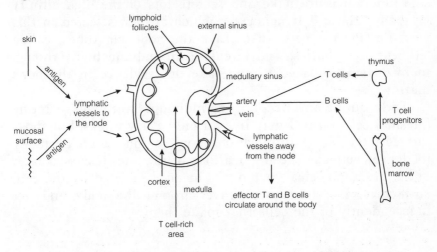

The meeting of foreign antigen with T and B lymphocytes results in their activation and differentiation to become effector T cells e.g. (TLS) or B cells (plasma cells), or memory T or B cells.

Immunocompetent but naive B and T cells travel from the bone marrow or the thymus to the node, and become localised in different parts of the node. Foreign material (protein, virus, bacterium, parasite) may enter the body due to a break either in the skin or at a mucosal surface. Some may travel directly via a lymph duct to the nearest lymph node or be taken up by a dendritic cell conveniently 'lying in wait' near the skin, and be similarly transported to the node. They enter the marginal (external) sinus (passage) which leads into the medulla (central part) where foreign antigen may be phagocytosed by macrophages lining the sinuses in the medulla. Antigen-containing dendritic cells make their way to the T cell rich area and interact with the T cells (discussed later).

Once activated, T helper cells may then travel to the cortex and interact there with B cells. Once this has happened, B cells migrate to the lymphoid follicles and undergo a process called 'affinity maturation'. Frequent mutations occur in the variable regions of the antibody molecule. Some of these result in the ability of an antibody molecule to bind with the antigen being considerably increased (affinity maturation). Those B cells which do this best are selected to become plasma cells whose sole function is to make and secrete lots of the high affinity antibody. Those B lymphocytes which are not selected in this way die. Plasma cells then leave the node via tubes, called 'efferent' lymphatics, and circulate around the body, though many plasma cells go to and take up residence in the bone marrow.

Early during an infection, the individual antibody-secreting (plasma) cells formed may live for only a few weeks, but those formed later during an infection may live and secrete antibody for longer periods. The implications of this are discussed later under 'immunological memory'. But once secreted by the cell, antibodies, like hormones, travel around the body and act independently of the cells that made them.

INTERACTION OF ANTIGEN WITH T LYMPHOCYTES

Whereas B lymphocytes directly bind an antigen, T lymphocytes react only indirectly with a foreign antigen—it has first to be processed by another cell (an antigen-presenting cell) to form smaller molecules, called peptides. These peptides are a linear sequence of between 9 to 25 amino acids in length. This peptide combines with a host protein molecule, called a major histocompatibility complex (MHC) antigen and it is this complex—

MHC/antigen/foreign peptide—which is recognised by a receptor on the T lymphocyte and leads to its activation and differentiation. How does this come about?

In the 1940s when Macfarlane Burnet was puzzling about tolerance—how the body distinguished between self and not-self, he proposed that cells and products in one individual's body would have a 'self-marker' which would distinguish them from 'foreign' products, for example, from somebody else's cells or from infected cells. He later discarded this idea as being too 'improbable'. It was later shown that the body achieved this distinction between self and not-self in quite a different way. Major histocompatibility complex antigens are highly polymorphic (meaning that they have many different shapes or structures), but an individual person has only a small number. In the 1950s, Peter Medawar (who shared the 1960 Nobel Prize with Burnet), published a book called *The Uniqueness of the Individual*, based on the fact that apart from identical twins, it was unlikely that two people would have exactly the same histocompatibility antigenic specificities. In humans, these antigens are called *H*uman *L*eucocyte *A*ntigens, or HLA). Table 4.3 outlines the basis of this polymorphism.

There are two classes of major histocompatibility complex molecules—class I and class II. Nearly every cell type in the body expresses the class I molecules on its surface. In contrast, the class II molecules are expressed mainly on cells which can act as antigen-presenting cells. They are 'strong' antigens, so if cells from one individual are transferred to another individual, as in a heart or kidney transplant, the immune system of the recipient recognises the foreign histocompatibility antigen on the cells. An immune response against it is then generated and the transplant is rejected (see Figure 4.1). This can be avoided if the immune system of the recipient is suppressed at the time of the transplant and for some time after that.

It was obvious that these histocompatibility antigens were not present on cells just to frustrate surgeons carrying out tissue transplantations; they must be there for some other reason to do with the immune system, but no-one knew why. The availability of inbred animals beginning from the late 1950s made it possible to investigate this question.

Table 4.3   The polymorphism of the major human MHC (HLA) antigens

Class	Chromosome	Loci	Number of alleles*
I	6	A	59
		B	111
		C	37
II	6	DPα	8
		DPβ	62
		DQα	16
		DQβ	25
		DRα	1
		DRβ	122

*   Molecules with different amino acid sequences which present different antigen fragments. Each class I MHC molecule consists of a single amino acid chain, complexed with a conserved molecule B2 microglobulin. In contrast, each class II MHC molecule has an α and β amino acid chain, so that the final molecule is, for example, DP αβ. As with antibodies, having two variable chains greatly increases the polymorphism (variability) that the complete molecule can express.

The figures quoted are reproduced with permission from C.A. Janeway and P. Travers (1997). *Immunobiology. The immune system in health and disease.* Current Biology Ltd, London.

The numbers quoted are minimal, and are mainly gained from Caucasian populations. Global figures including all populations would be considerably larger.

Each embryo at conception receives genes coding for one allele at each genetic locus from each parent. The overall pattern so obtained is called a haplotype. Thus each person has two specificities (alleles) at the loci, A, B, C, DP, DQ and DR. Because of the very large number of alleles, the total possible number of different haplotypes is literally enormous, and this is why each individual, other than identical twins, is likely to have a unique haplotype. The composition of the haplotype determines the likelihood of a strong, reasonable or poor immune response by T cells to an infection, and especially to some vaccines. Examples are given in Chapter 5.

As with antibodies, the variation in specificity of an MHC molecule occurs in a small region, the variable region, thus limiting the amount of DNA coding for MHC molecules.

THE ROLE OF MAJOR HISTOCOMPATIBILITY COMPLEX (MHC) ANTIGENS

It had been known for many years that to induce a strong antibody production to a foreign protein in outbred rabbits, i.e., bred by random mating so that each individual was unique (like humans), one should immunise 4 or 5 animals. A couple might make strong responses, another couple weaker responses and one might make very little antibody. Baruj Benacerraf (USA) used two inbred strains of guinea pigs (bred by repeated brother/sister mating). All the members of each strain were genetically identical. When he immunised these in an identical fashion in the early 1960s, all the animals in *each* strain were shown to make very similar responses, but the mean antibody level in one strain was much higher than that of the other strain. This showed that the immune response was genetically controlled and the genes involved were labelled Ir (immune response) genes. Benacerraf shared the 1980 Nobel Prize for this and other related findings. In the mid-1960s while working in London, Hugh McDevitt (USA) and colleagues made similar findings in inbred strains of mice shortly thereafter. In this case, it became even more clearcut because strains could be bred in which the only difference was their histocompatibility antigen specificities.

In the late 1960s, it was found that one type of T cell (which came to be called a cytotoxic or 'killer' T lymphocyte, commonly shortened to CTL) from a mouse (A) which had been injected with cells from another mouse strain (B) which differed mainly in their histocompatibility antigen specificities, could, in a test tube, lyse (kill) cells from the B mouse strain. In the late 1960s, Robert Blanden in the John Curtin School of Medical Research at the Australian National University in Canberra showed that if mice were injected with a potentially lethal dose of a poxvirus, ectromelia (mousepox virus), transfer of T cells from a mouse of the same strain which had recovered from this infection protected the mice from death. Transfer of specific immune serum had a much less protective effect. He later showed that the cells involved possessed cytotoxic (killer) activity because if they were added to cells infected with this virus—these 'target' cells were from mice of the same strain— these infected target cells were lysed (killed). Uninfected cells were not killed. Importantly, the infected cells were killed before viral progeny was made, thus explaining how T cells controlled the viral infection. Bob Blanden was also collaborating with Hugh McDevitt (USA) on the puzzle—how does possession of some histocompatibility genes in mice confer strong resistance to mousepox virus infection?

In the early 1970s, two young scientists in the same department (Microbiology) in the John Curtin School now became interested—Peter Doherty, an Australian, and Rolf Zinkernagel, a visitor from Switzerland. They worked with a different virus, lymphocytic choriomeningitis virus (LCMV) in mice. Both ectromelia (mousepox) and LCM viruses are natural pathogens of mice. Doherty and Zinkernagel asked a simple question—if cytotoxic T lymphocytes from strain A mice could kill LCM virus-infected cells (called target cells) from strain A mice, would they also kill LCM virus-infected target cells from a different mouse strain, B? The major histocompatibility complex antigens of strains A and B mice were of quite different specificities. The answer was completely clearcut—no! The reverse experiment gave a similar answer—cytotoxic T lymphocytes from strain B LCM virus-infected mice (strain B) killed LCM virus-infected strain B infected target cells, but not strain A LCM virus-infected cells. They then showed that if mice of the different strains shared only a single histocompatibility antigen specificity, this killing would still occur. In a brief article in the British journal, the *Lancet*, they proposed that the role of the major histocompatibility complex antigens was to combine with an antigen from the virus infecting the cell and that this combination, presented at the infected cell surface, was recognised as 'foreign' by the T cell receptor. The role of the major histocompatibility complex molecule was to signal to the immune system a change in the antigenicity of the cell.

Over the next 20 years, it was found initially by Emil Unanue (USA) that it was a peptide derived from a foreign, ingested antigen (not the intact antigen itself) which bound to the class II histocompatibility antigen. Alain Townsend (UK) later showed that a peptide from a newly synthesised viral antigen bound to the class I histocompatibility antigen. Generally, this latter peptide is about 9 amino acids (range, 8–10 amino acids) in length, and hence is called a nonamer. Pam Bjorkman, Jack Strominger and Don Wiley with colleagues (USA) were able to crystallise the peptide/major histocompatibility antigen complex and showed that the peptide was held in a groove at the tip of the major histocompatibility complex molecule. Thus, it became clear that the T cell receptor recognised an 'area' of the complex which contained both the peptide and the tip of the histocompatibility molecule. (The mechanism of this binding is discussed in more detail in Chapter 5). In 1995, Doherty, Zinkernagel, Unanue, Strominger and Wiley shared the Lasker Award (the most prestigious award for biomedical research in the USA), and in 1996, Zinkernagel and Doherty were awarded the Nobel Prize in Physiology or Medicine in recognition of their original discovery of the role of the major histocompatibility complex (MHC) antigens in immune recognition.

In his view of how the immune system worked, Burnet had earlier used the terms, self and not-self, but Zinkernagel and Doherty had now added an extra term, altered self. The distinction was as follows:

self—self MHC molecule complexed with a peptide from a cell protein of the same host;

not-self—a foreign MHC molecule and peptide also from the unrelated host, e.g. in a grafted tissue;

altered self—self MHC molecule complexed with a peptide from an invading infectious agent—virus, bacterium or parasite.

Zinkernagel and Doherty also coined the phrase that cytotoxic T lymphocyte (CTL) activity was *MHC-restricted*, to indicate the dominant role played by the MHC molecule in antigen presentation. In every case, class I MHC molecules were involved and the peptide, foreign or self, had to be derived from a protein synthesised in the cell.

By this time, it was known that there were two main classes of T lymphocytes. One type expressed a cell membrane marker called CD4 and were thus called CD4 positive; the other class expressed the cell marker CD8 (CD8 positive lymphocytes). In each case these markers are adjacent to and helped to stabilise the T cell receptor. Lymphocytes with cytotoxic activity expressed the CD8 marker. As well as having cytotoxic activity, these CD8+ lymphocytes secreted a number of cytokines, including gamma interferon, and some chemokines. Because class I histocompatibility molecules are expressed on nearly every cell type in the body, effector T lymphocytes possessing cytotoxic activity are potentially the major mechanism for controlling infection (by killing infected cells) once infection of a host occurs.

In contrast, class II histocompatibility molecules are expressed mainly on cells which can act as antigen-presenting cells (APCs). In this case, non-infectious proteins or particles can be ingested (phagocytosed) by an APC and these are degraded to peptides by enzymes in structures called lysosomes. Some of these, average length about 15 amino acids, can combine with a class II histocompatibility molecule and the complex be presented at the surface of the APC. The receptors of CD4+ T lymphocytes recognise this class II MHC/peptide complex on the APC.

Kevin Lafferty, also working in the John Curtin School in Canberra in the early 1970s, showed for the first time that in order to induce a response by a T lymphocyte, the APC must also express on their surface a molecule, called a co-stimulator, which is also recognised by the CD4+T lymphocyte. This dual recognition of antigen and co-stimulator activates the T lymphocyte and initiates its differentiation. One of two events can happen. It can become a Type 1 CD4+ T lymphocyte that makes a range of cytokines similar to those made by cytotoxic lymphocytes, but it can also 'help' the latter to mature and some B cells to make IgG antibodies. Or it can become a Type 2 CD4+ T lymphocyte which makes quite a different pattern of cytokines. Their only or major role is to 'help' B cells to become plasma cells and make IgG, IgA or IgE.

At present, it is clear that there are two 'dominant' cytokines. Production of interleukin 4 (IL–4) favours the induction of a Type 2 T lymphocyte response, resulting in production of mainly antibodies, and can down-regulate a type 1 T cell response. In contrast, production of interleukin–12 (IL–12) favours a Type 1 T lymphocyte response. A recent case report of a three-year girl who had recurrent bacterial infections showed that the patient suffered a profound deficiency in the production of IL–12 (Haraguchi et al. 1998).

THE ROLE OF THE DIFFERENT IMMUNE RESPONSES IN PREVENTING, CONTROLLING AND CLEARING AN INTRACELLULAR INFECTION

This is summarised in Table 4.4. The major message of the table is the *complementary roles* of antibody and T lymphocytes, particularly the CD8+ cytotoxic T lymphocyte. A major role for antibody is to minimise or hopefully prevent infection, by 'neutralising' the infectivity of virus or bacterium, that is, preventing the agent from infecting a cell. In contrast, the major role of the T lymphocytes is to control and clear an infection once this has happened. This is elaborated further when discussing the sequence of events during an infection in a 'naive' (as compared to a specifically vaccinated) host—see Figure 4.4.

Many bacteria and parasites replicate outside cells in the body—called an extracellular infection. Here, antibody is responsible for both prevention and clearing the infection. Cytotoxic T cells would usually not be formed in this case, but CD4+ T lymphocytes would be formed because dead bacteria or antigen: antibody complexes would be ingested by phagocytic cells.

IMMUNOLOGICAL MEMORY

Like specificity, memory is a crucial property of the adaptive immune system. Without immunological memory, probably few of us would be alive today and vaccines wouldn't work! Even though the following description is a marked simplification of what we already know about immunological memory, there is still a lot we do not know.

When immunologically competent B lymphocytes are activated following exposure to antigen, they become plasma cells whose sole task is to make and secrete lots of antibody. Many plasma cells only live for a few weeks so there has to be a way to ensure the continuing production of antibody. This is achieved by some cells becoming only 'partly activated' but persisting for a long time. They are called memory B cells and they continually circulate around the body. After the initial infection, some of the antigen from the virus/bacteria can persist for a very long time at a special site (lymphoid follicles) in the lymphoid tissues (Figure 4.3). When a memory B cell circulates through a lymph node again, it may contact this

Table 4.4   A summary of the roles of antibody and different T cells in preventing, controlling or clearing an intracellular infection

Immune response	Role before/during an infection		
	Preventing	Controlling	Clearing
Antibody (B lymphocytes)	+++	+	+
CD4+ Th2 cells	–	–	–
CD4+ Th1 cells	–	+	+
CD8+ CTLs	–	+	+++

+++ Very important; ++ Important; + Minor role; – No direct role depot of antigen and if so, it is easily converted to a plasma cell. As a result, much more of the same antibody is made. The net result of this process is that after an initial infection, specific antibody is continually made, sometimes for very long periods (decades). The continual presence of this antibody is very likely to protect a person from disease caused by a second similar infection (Table 4.4).

As well as the early comments of Thucydides about protection from a second attack of the plague, there are historical examples involving people in isolated communities such as the Faroe Islands north of Scotland who survived a first measles infection. They were protected from a second infection when measles reached the islands again about 50 years later. In contrast, those not born at the time of the first infection were infected the second time around. Generally, vaccines are not as efficient as the natural infection at inducing long-lived protection after a single exposure. Two or more administrations of the vaccines are often required to induce persisting antibody production, but this is a small price to pay for the safer protection given by the vaccine.

Activation and differentiation of T lymphocytes yields a population of memory cells as well as effector lymphocytes, such as those with cytotoxic activity. These memory cells are both more readily and more rapidly activated to become effector cells compared to their precursor (naive) cells. The memory cells can live a very long time, possibly the life of the host. But they are usually not activated until there is another exposure to the same (or a similar) infectious agent that caused their formation originally.

Both infection and vaccination result in a substantial increase in the number of both types of memory cells, relative to the original number of naive precursor cells.

The sequence of immune responses during an intracellular infection

The pattern seen during infection in a model system is shown in Figure 4.4. In this case, mice were infected with influenza virus which then replicates in the lung. The lungs were measured, at different times (varying from days to months) after the infection, for levels of:

- infectious virus;
- cytotoxic T lymphocyte (CTL) activity;
- specific antibody secreting cells (ASCs);
- memory CTLs and *memory* ASCs.

The important results were as follows:

1   The level of infectious virus initially increases and then falls so that infectious virus is no longer detectable after about ten days. The fall in virus level coincides closely with the increase in cytotoxic T lymphocyte activity.
2   This cytotoxic activity disappears about four days after infectious virus is no longer detectable. That is, infected cells are necessary to stimulate CD8+ T lymphocytes to become cytotoxic effector cells which once formed, have a rather short life. High levels of memory CD8+ Lymphocytes are found at about two weeks after infection. Additional experiments indicate high levels of these memory cells may persist for at least 18 months.
3   Antibody-secreting cells are constantly present from about 7–8 days until at least 18 months, indicating that antibody is constantly being produced. Memory B cells reach their highest level at about two months after the initiation of infection.

This is the usual pattern of responses to an infection, but it may be much more drawn out. During human HIV infection for example, a strong viraemia (lots of free infectious virus in the blood) sometimes occurs at about three weeks after infection. Cellular cytotoxic activity is detected at this time and this coincides with a great decrease (but not a complete disappearance) in the virus level in the blood. Infectivity-neutralising antibody is often not detected until some weeks later.

The general findings indicate that the cytotoxic T lymphocyte response rather than neutralising antibody, is the first main adaptive immune mechanism to appear after an intracellular infection has begun and which can control or clear the infection.

Vaccination

The pattern seen following vaccination with a live, attenuated viral vaccine will in principle be similar to that seen following

**Figure 4.4   The sequence of two immune responses, cytotoxic T
lymphocyte activity and specific antibody-secreting cells,
in the lungs of mice following an influenza virus infection**

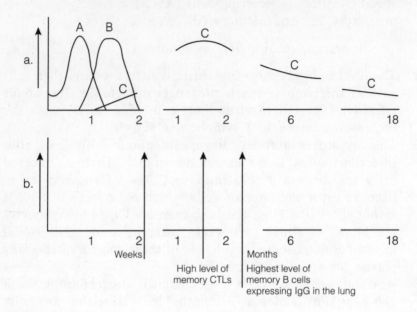

Graph a
Vertical axis: level of infectious virus in the lungs, and effector T and B lymphocyte activity following virus administration.
Horizontal axis: time (days, weeks, months) after administration of influenza virus
Curves: A, infectious influenza virus; B, specific cytotoxic T lymphocyte (CTL) activity; C, specific antibody-secreting cell (ASC) levels.
Graph b
Times after infection when high levels of memory CTLs and of specific memory B cells were found. Note that CTL activity is present for a relatively short period after infection, but by about two weeks, there are many memory CTLs. In contrast, ASCs are continually present after about 1 week, thus ensuring the constant presence of antibody so that a second infection by the same virus would be prevented.

Reproduced with permission from Gordon Ada and Alastair Ramsay (1997) *Vaccines, Vaccination and the Immune Response*. Lippincott-Raven Press, Philadelphia.

the natural infection. Vaccination with an inactivated or a subunit preparation should result in a basically similar pattern of antibody production, but although CD4+ T lymphocyte responses would be seen, production of CD8+ cytotoxic T lymphocytes most likely would be absent as their production usually depends upon active infection of the antigen-presenting cell.

The great majority of current vaccines (Chapter 3) are against viruses or bacteria which show little antigenic variation

The main solution sought by vaccine developers has been to induce an antibody response which is of the correct specificity and is so strong that upon later exposure to the natural infectious agent, almost all of the infectious agent is neutralised. The amount which escapes to infect the host is so small that it would induce only a 'subclinical' infection (that is, one in which there is no sign of disease).

The main exception to this situation is the influenza virus which does show significant antigenic variation. Vaccine developers combat this by making a new vaccine every year, matching as far as is possible the antigenic pattern of recently circulating strains.

In this chapter, we have mainly discussed the way the adaptive immune response works. It is an extraordinarily complex but wonderfully orchestrated response and many of the details have become clear only recently. The main characteristics of this system are specificity and long-lived memory, and successful vaccine development is utterly dependent upon these factors. The two major effector responses are humoral (antibody production) and cell-mediated (differentiated T lymphocytes). The major role of antibody is to prevent (neutralise) or greatly minimise the infectivity of the infecting agent, and vaccine manufacturers have understandably made the achievement of this type of immune response their major goal. This becomes more difficult to achieve if the infectious agent shows great antigenic variation, as occurs with agents such as HIV, malaria and chlamydia. Making candidate vaccines to these agents based solely on an antibody approach has had only limited success to date. The newer approaches to vaccine design for these diseases increasingly depend upon inducing a strong cell-mediated immune response, including cytotoxic T lymphocyte induction, and this is discussed in Chapter 10.

5

Vaccine efficacy and the variation in individual responses

In order to be licensed for human use, a vaccine must be demonstrated to be effective. The basic criterion of vaccine efficacy is that if the vaccinated individual is later exposed to the natural infectious agent, disease does not occur. This does not mean that infection will not occur. In fact, it could be argued that a very mild infection after vaccination could boost the level of protection given by the vaccine, and this probably happens frequently. However, the desired effect is that once exposed, the person previously vaccinated has at the most a subclinical infection, does not suffer any illness and does not pass on the infection to others who may not have been vaccinated, such as, younger siblings. Once some experience has been gained with a vaccine's use, an indication of its efficacy can be gained by measuring specific antibody levels at different times after administration of the vaccine.

Once vaccines have been used for some time and the incidence of disease has fallen sharply, people's memories of the clinical disease caused by the natural agent in the population start to fade, and concern about adverse side effects following vaccination grows. The way to get a more balanced view is to consider data on the efficacy of vaccines on disease incidence over time, and compare recent levels with the levels for some years before vaccination was introduced. Such information is provided in this chapter.

Figure 5.1 **Whooping cough notifications; cases and deaths in England and Wales from 1940 to 1973. Mass vaccination was introduced during 1950–1957. This is part of the graph which is reproduced in full in Figure 6.2.**

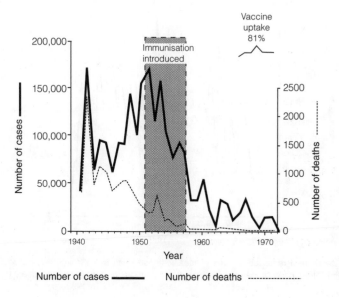

LEARNING FROM EPIDEMICS

Before vaccines became available, disease due to infections was widespread and usually occurred in a series of 'waves' or epidemics. Some epidemics of great historic importance were mentioned in Chapter 1.

Figure 5.1 shows the number of notifications of cases of whooping cough in England and Wales from 1940, until vaccination was introduced in 1950 and the levels reached by the early 1970s when vaccine coverage had reached 81 per cent. Between 1941 and the early 1950s the annual incidence of cases was always above 50,000, with maximum levels reaching 150,000 to 170,000 cases per year. As a result of the introduction of mass immunisation, there was a dramatic reduction in the number of both cases and deaths. On three occasions between 1962 and 1972, the annual number of cases was less than 15,000. After that time, an unfortunate event happened which is described in the next chapter.

Figure 5.2   Reported cases of measles each year in the USA from 1912 to 1966, and at three times after 1966. Mass immunisation against measles was initiated in 1963.

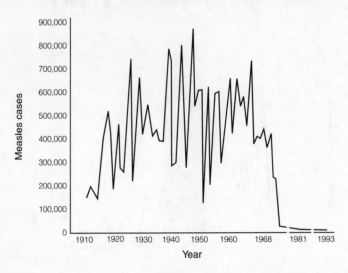

Note: The highest recorded number of measles cases was 894,134 in 1941, but following the introduction of mass immunisation, the number of cases reported decreased rapidly, to 22,231 in 1968, to 3,124 in 1981 and to 312 in 1993.

Figure 5.2 shows the incidence of cases of measles in the USA from 1912 to 1963 when the first measles vaccine was introduced. During this time the population of the USA almost doubled in size, from 95 to 188 million and there was a series of major epidemics, which on several occasions reached nearly 900,000 cases. Furthermore, some epidemics occurred only two or three years apart. Mass immunisation was introduced in 1963 and the annual number of cases fell from 458,000 in 1964 to 22,000 in 1968. That is a drop of more than 95 per cent in four years.

A similar pattern of 'peaks and valleys', with levels varying between about 180,000 and 800,000 cases a year in the incidence of measles, was observed in England and Wales from 1941 to 1968. When mass immunisation was introduced in 1968, the incidence of clinical infections dropped significantly within a few years—similar to the experience with whooping cough.

Epidemics are most clearly seen with agents which are highly infectious via the respiratory or oral route. When one epidemic has passed, there is a gradual build-up of susceptible but uninfected individuals with the result that the level of herd immunity significantly decreases. (Herd immunity is the level of immunity in the population which occurs when a sufficiently high proportion of susceptible people have been immunised. Transmission from person to person stops so that no new cases occur.) However, once the level of herd immunity decreases to a sufficiently low level, another epidemic can occur. The level of 'protective' herd immunity with measles is very high, about 95 per cent. Reduction of only a few per cent could allow an epidemic to occur.

Disease due to vector-borne infectious agents may also show a similar pattern. Dengue fever (a mosquito-borne disease) has been endemic in tropical countries in the Western Pacific region for many years, and there have been regular epidemics. The disease was initially confined to this region, but with increasing urbanisation and rapid air travel, dengue haemorrhagic fever has spread in epidemics to west Asia, the Pacific islands and to the Americas. In 1917, there was an outbreak of encephalitis in the Murray Valley region in Australia, but the agent was not identified. There was another major epidemic in 1951, and the virus was then isolated and characterised for the first time. Because of its novel properties, it was called Murray River encephalitis virus. The reason for this second outbreak was a very wet period in eastern Australia in the months preceding the epidemic, allowing the migration of infected birds (the natural hosts) from North Australia down the Darling River in western New South Wales, and into the Murray River Valley. Local mosquitoes feeding on these birds became infected and in turn infected humans in this general area—hence the name given to the disease.

In contrast, some infections don't show this pattern of epidemics. Tetanus infection is not naturally transmissible between infected people. In the USA, there was a steady decline of tetanus infections since the introduction of the vaccine in the early 1940s. Notifications were 560 cases in 1947 and 27 cases in 1996. The major cause for concern now is the very high rate of neonatal tetanus infection in many Third World countries due to unhygienic birthing practices, such as putting mud on the umbilical stump after the cord is cut. Such practices result in infection and often death especially of the newborn.

VACCINE EFFICACY

In the USA, the Centers for Disease Control and Prevention (CDC, Atlanta, Georgia) have recorded each year the number of cases of different childhood infections occurring in the USA from as long ago as 1912 until the present day. It is an invaluable source of data of a kind not available in most countries. To indicate the efficacy of vaccines the levels during a major epidemic before vaccines became available and those in recent years, in most cases many years after the introduction of a specific vaccine, have been compared.

Table 5.1 compares the incidence of cases in the USA of infection by common childhood infectious agents during a major epidemic before the vaccine became available with the number of cases in 1992 and 1996. In most cases, this is well after the vaccine first became available. The introduction of compulsory vaccination in the USA had a marked beneficial effect. To drive home the remarkable achievements of vaccination in controlling these diseases, these figures of over 99 per cent reduction in incidence of disease cases can be viewed in a different way, as follows:

Imagine that in one year, nearly everybody in a *city* (about 1 million population) was sick with measles; now, after the introduction of vaccination, only the people living in one small *street* in the city are sick.

Imagine that in the past about two out of every three people in a city (about 300,000 population) in any one year had diphtheria; now only one person in that city has this infection each year.

Imagine that once everyone in a large suburb (about 25,000 population) of a city had paralytic poliomyelitis; now, nobody in that suburb has that disease!

The results with pertussis (whooping cough) are not quite so dramatic, but a decrease in incidence of over 97 per cent is still a remarkable achievement! A possible reason for this lower value of efficacy is the recent indication from European experiences that some batches of the pertussis vaccine may be less effective than others. The replacement of the whole cell vaccine by acellular (subunit) preparations should remedy this situation.

The Australian data with *Haemophilus influenzae* type b (Hib) vaccination shows a very large drop (about 90 per cent)

Table 5.1   Vaccine efficacy (per cent decrease in incidence of different infectious diseases) in the USA, as assessed by comparing maximum morbidity levels (before vaccine availability) and the levels some years after compulsory vaccination was introduced

	Before vaccination		After vaccination		% decrease in disease
	No. of cases	Year	No. of cases in		incidence*
			1992	1996	
Diphtheria	206,919	1921 (1942)**	4	1	99.99
Measles	894,134	1941 (1963)	2,237	500	99.95
Mumps	152,209	1968 (1971)	2,572	600	99.60
Rubella	57,686	1969 (1971)	160	210	99.64
Pertussis	265,269	1934 (1945)	4,083	6,400	97.6
Polio (paralytic)	21,269	1952 (1952)	4	0	100.00
(total)	57,879				
Haemophilus influenzae type b (Hib)	20,000	1984 (1987)	1,412	1,065	94.68

Data kindly supplied by Drs W. Orenstein and R. Bernstein, Centers for Disease Control and Prevention, Atlanta.

*   Calculation based on 1996 figures.

**   Dates in parenthesis indicate the year the vaccine was generally introduced. MMR vaccine was introduced in 1971. IPV (Salk) vaccine was introduced in 1952 and OPV (Sabin) vaccine in 1963.

in incidence of disease within two years (1993–1995) of the introduction of vaccination (Figure 5.3). The control of this infection should continue to improve in the next few years.

Measles is an important case for discussion because of its very high transmission rates. As seen from Figure 5.2, the incidence of cases in the USA was always above 100,000 per year prior to the introduction of the vaccine. It fell from over 458,000 cases in 1964 to less than 22,000 cases in 1968 and by 1981, the number of cases was less than 10,000 per year for the first time. It remained low (less than 4,000 cases) until 1988 when there was an epidemic lasting for three years, during which the incidence of cases nearly reached 28,000 in 1990. This epidemic was due to two main factors. Vaccination coverage in depressed inner areas of some large cities was not maintained and importantly, it was realised that a two-dose vaccination schedule was required to fully prevent outbreaks of this infection. Since these deficiencies were corrected, the level of cases decreased to a record low in 1997 when only

Figure 5.3   Notifications by age groups of *Haemophilus influenzae* type b (Hib) in Australia from January 1951 to March 1995. The vaccine was introduced during 1992.

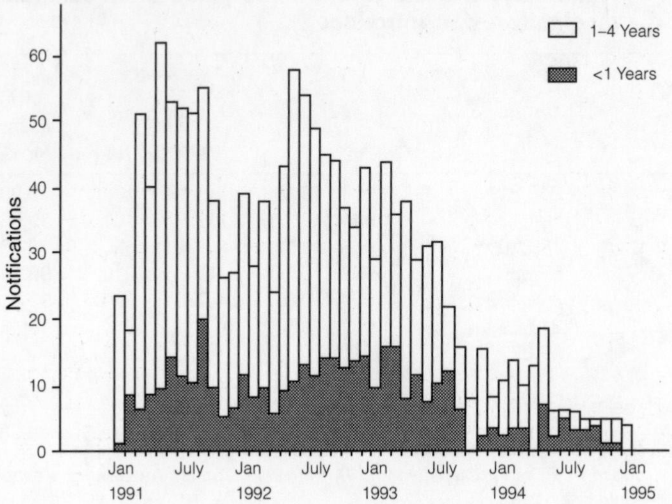

Reproduced with permission from Gordon Ada and Alastair Ramsay (1997). *Vaccines, Vaccination and the Immune Response*. Lippincott-Raven Press, Philadelphia.

135 cases were detected. It has since been established that these cases were all imported, indicating that natural transmission of measles infection within the USA had been prevented— a remarkable achievement.

In 1998, a special two-dose measles immunisation programme was instituted in Australia because of the real concern that an epidemic was likely to occur, as had been the recent experience in New Zealand.

Over the years, it has been the general experience that the introduction of a vaccine against a current infectious disease and its widespread use has resulted in a rapid and significant decrease in the incidence of disease cases.

On the other hand, a breakdown in vaccine availability can rapidly result in an outbreak of infectious disease. There were major outbreaks of diseases such as diphtheria in parts of the former USSR following the disintegration of the Republic. The 800 cases of diphtheria reported in 1989 had risen to more than 50,000 by 1994. Diphtheria is now endemic in Algeria and as the country slides towards civil war, prospects for containment are grim. A similar situation occurred in the former Yugoslavia when hostilities broke out and the vaccine supply chain broke down. Globally, the prevalence of that ancient scourge, the plague (*Yersinia pestis*) has increased sixfold in the past 15 years. Occasional cases have been reported in the USA, but the disease is endemic in Burma and South Vietnam.

Do improvements in health as well as in personal and community hygiene result in a lower incidence of infectious diseases?

This certainly can happen! The availability of adequate water supplies and the virtual absence of severe malnutrition in industrialised countries has resulted in the almost complete disappearance of cholera infections in those countries. On the other hand, there are regular outbreaks of cholera in some developing countries, especially when those fleeing from local hostilities are herded together in temporary camps with inadequate water and food supplies. Globally, about 150,000 cases were diagnosed in 1996.

Leprosy—also known as Hansen's disease—was rife in Europe early this century but has now almost disappeared from that region. It remains a serious disease of millions of people in countries like India and of disadvantaged groups of people such as the Australian Aborigines. Attempts to make an effective vaccine to control leprosy have so far been largely unsuccessful, but there is now increasing hope that it can be controlled by chemotherapy. Compared to measles, leprosy is a rather poorly infectious disease.

The situation is quite different with highly infectious diseases. It is great for a child to be healthy and well fed, but this may induce in the parents a sense of false security against infectious diseases, as will be discussed in the rest of this chapter.

The incidence early in the 1990s of two highly infectious viral diseases for which vaccines were not then available

Rotavirus and respiratory syncytial viruses are highly infectious pathogens and cause childhood diarrhoea and respiratory infections respectively. Worldwide, diarrhoea is at the top of the list of major killers (Table 1.3) with most deaths occurring in developing countries. Rotavirus is the leading cause of severe diarrhoeal disease in infants in both developed and developing countries. Before the age of 5, over 80 per cent of children in the USA and over 90 per cent in the developing countries will experience at least one rotavirus infection, resulting in diarrhoea. The incidence of moderate to severe cases is about 12.5 per cent in both regions. In other words, the superior living conditions and children's generally good health in the USA does not prevent rotavirus infection leading to either mild or severe disease. The introduction of a rotavirus vaccine in the USA in 1998 should have a marked effect on the incidence of the disease in that country, and results should become apparent early in the new millennium.

Respiratory syncytial virus (RSV) is the single most important cause of severe lower respiratory tract infections in infants and young children. It is a common cause of winter outbreaks of acute respiratory disease and in the USA, results in an estimated 90,000 hospitalisations and 4,500 deaths each year. The global annual infection and mortality figures for RSV are estimated to be 64 million and 160,000 respectively. There can be repeated infections throughout life. Nearly all children are infected by 2 years of age. Infections later in life cause milder disease. Attempts to make a vaccine started in the 1960s, but it is only comparatively recently that some more encouraging results have been obtained.

THE GLOBAL PREVALENCE OF SOME SEXUALLY TRANSMITTED DISEASES

More than 30 bacterial, viral and parasitic diseases have now been identified that can be transmitted by the sexual route. The greatest risk of infection is in sexually active individuals and infants born to infected mothers. Multiple infections within the same individual are common. In 1995, the global total of *new cases* of four (curable) diseases, gonorrhoea, chlamydia, syphilis and trichomoniasis, was 333 million, including Australasia, 1 million; North America, 14 million; and Western Europe, 16 million.

INDIVIDUAL RESPONSES TO DIFFERENT VACCINES

As explained in Chapter 4, the immune response is genetically determined at the level of the T cell. The T cell receptor recognises a complex between the major histocompatibility complex (MHC) molecule and the peptide derived from the foreign antigen. This is illustrated in Figure 5.4. Because of the restricted size of the peptide involved (it is a nonamer, i.e., nine amino acids in length), it is simplest to consider first the activation of CD8+ T lymphocytes to become effector cells and have cytotoxic activity. The cells are then called cytotoxic T lymphocytes (CTLs).

As was done in Chapter 4, we first provide a condensed and simplified version of why an individual responds differently to different vaccines. This is then followed by the more detailed version.

Part 1—A summary of the main points

1 MHC antigens are an extremely variable family of proteins (Table 4.3). Each individual has a very small selection of the total and this grouping is unique to that individual.

2 In order to complex with a particular MHC molecule, a peptide must have particular properties such as the sequence of amino acids. If several of all the nonapeptides in the proteins of say, a virus, bind well to an individual's set of MHC proteins, a good immune response will be made to that virus. As the number which bind well decreases, the immune response is likely to become weaker.

3 If none bind, the individual will not respond to the vaccine. Ten–15 per cent of adult recipients of the subunit hepatitis B vaccine respond poorly or not at all. This can be 'corrected' by adding extra special peptides (T cell epitopes) to the vaccine.

4 An immunologically normal individual (child, adult) is likely to respond well to most vaccines but less well to the others. The latter vaccines are unlikely to protect that individual completely from a later infection by that agent. However, *if not vaccinated*, they may become very sick or even die if later exposed to that infectious agent. It is much safer to be vaccinated!

Figure 5.4   **A diagrammatic representation of the recognition by the cytotoxic T lymphocyte (CTL) receptor of the complex between the MHC molecule and the nonapeptide (T cell epitope) on the surface of the antigen-presenting cell (APC).**

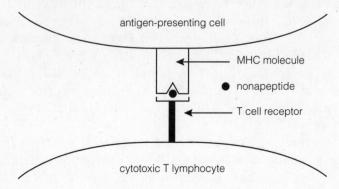

5   Predicting those infectious diseases to which an individual may be highly susceptible is not yet feasible. However, data is now available which strongly suggests that having genes coding for certain class I MHC specificities protects those individuals from very serious effects of infections such as HIV, malaria and chlamydia (see Chapter 10).

Part 2—A more detailed explanation

THE BASIC REQUIREMENTS FOR RECOGNITION OF ANTIGENS BY T LYMPHOCYTES

There are two basic requirements for recognition of antigens which can then contribute to T lymphocyte activation. First, the peptide must combine with the MHC (in humans, called HLA, but we will often use the general term, MHC or major histocompatibility proteins) molecule with a sufficient affinity to form a stable complex. A protein with a linear sequence of say 60 amino acids will contain many nonamers—amino acids sequences 1–9, 2–10, 3–11 etc. up to 51–60 are all nonamers. However, only a tiny fraction, if any, of those in a particular foreign protein will bind with sufficient affinity to a protein encoded by a host's class I MHC gene. (The reader's memory about the tremendous polymorphism, i.e., variability, of MHC proteins may need to be refreshed by looking again at Table 4.3). One peptide may bind to say one particular class I MHC protein but not to any other class I MHC protein in that human host. The main reason is that in order for this binding to occur, particular amino acids must occupy usually two positions, but sometimes only one position, in the nonamer, usually positions close to each end. Different amino acids in some other positions can also influence the binding affinity. Furthermore, to be effective, the peptide-MHC complex once formed should be stable for some time, probably for several days.

Secondly, the peptide-MHC complex on the antigen-presenting cell (APC) has to be recognised by and bind with sufficient affinity to the receptor on an individual's CD8+ T lymphocyte in order to initiate the process of activation of that T cell. Figure 5.4 illustrates the binding of the peptide-MHC complex on the surface of the APC with the receptor on the T lymphocyte.

THE FREQUENCY OF OCCURRENCE OF APPROPRIATE T CELL EPITOPES IN VIRAL ANTIGENS

For any one individual, these conditions are very demanding. For person A, there may be only very few (if any) appropriate nonamers in the proteins of an average sized virus particle which would bind to one or more of his or her class I MHC proteins. There may be more for person B. Fortunately, some proteins are richer sources of effective nonamers, commonly called T cell epitopes, than others. For example, the nucleoprotein, one of the eight proteins in the influenza virus, and which is associated with the nucleic acid in the virus particle, contains different nonamers which bind well to a range of class I MHC proteins.

Generally, the same type of restrictions apply to peptides which bind to class II MHC proteins; in this case, the binding peptide is much larger (average length, 15 amino acids) and may be longer than 20 amino acids in length. Type 2 T cells which recognise class II MHC-peptide complexes help B lymphocytes to switch to the production of IgG antibodies (IgG is a major class of antibody). About 95 per cent of recipients make protective levels of infectivity-neutralising antibody (IgG) to a single dose of measles vaccine, and about 99 per cent respond to two doses of the same vaccine. The measles virus contains six virus-specified different proteins so this result shows that there are sufficient T cell epitopes in the viral proteins which will bind to at least one class II MHC protein in Caucasians. Thus, an advantage of whole organism vaccines, whether viral or bacterial, is the high probability that there are sufficient proteins to provide a wide range of T cell epitopes so that most recipients (over 90 per cent) will make protective levels of neutralising antibody. There will be a proportion (less than 10 per cent) who will not be completely protected from disease when later exposed to the wild-type (natural) agent. But in these individuals, the subsequent infection will be much milder and less hazardous compared to an infection in an unvaccinated individual. The reason for this is that the vaccination, though it appears to fail in such individuals, actually primes the immune system so that a stronger response is made when the natural virus infection subsequently occurs.

Again, some viral proteins such as the 'core' protein of the hepatitis B virus, are a good source of helper T cell epitopes. It has also been found in studies with mice that some helper T cell epitopes can bind to a number of different class II MHC proteins, and they have been called 'universal' T cell epitopes. The extent to which such epitopes may be useful in facilitating the design of peptide-based vaccines for human use is not yet clear.

IMPROVING THE HEPATITIS B VIRAL VACCINE

Two other implications arise from this situation. Because of the potential great safety of subunit vaccines and following the general success of the hepatitis B surface antigen (HBsAg) vaccine (the first genetically engineered vaccine, see Chapter 2), this approach has been tried repeatedly in recent years to develop vaccines against other viruses, such as human immuno-deficiency virus (HIV) and respiratory syncytial virus (RSV). So far, these attempts have not been very successful. But it has also since become clear that the hepatitis B vaccine itself can be improved. Up to about 15 per cent of adult humans respond poorly or not at all to this vaccine. When given to different inbred strains of mice, it was found that mice from many strains responded very well but mice from a few other strains completely failed to respond. It was established that the reason for this non-responsiveness was the absence of T cell epitopes in the vaccine which reacted well with the class II MHC proteins of the non-responding mice. This unresponsiveness has now been remedied by adding to the vaccine several additional T cell epitopes, in the form of other peptides (T cell epitopes) from the hepatitis B virus. In the case of humans, the non-responders frequently express the class II major histocompatibility proteins, DR3 and DR7. Some recent versions of this vaccine contain these additional epitopes so that they should induce a higher proportion of people to respond to the vaccine. This experience with the hepatitis B viral vaccine illustrates a potential difficulty facing vaccine manufacturers who wish to develop these simpler forms of vaccines.

THE MESSAGE

The reason for going into the above detail is to illustrate two important points:

1   while all licensed human vaccines are effective, some can protect a higher proportion of recipients than others;
2   it is also to be expected that while a given individual will respond very well to most vaccines, he or she will respond less well to one or two other vaccines.

Put simply, a person is unlikely to possess the best set of MHC genes to respond with the highest efficiency to *all* infections. The situation will vary between different individuals. Sometimes, statements are made by a parent concerned about the safety of vaccines, like 'my two-year-old son or daughter is so healthy and well fed that he or she does not need to be vaccinated'. This is an irresponsible attitude by the parent who knows nothing about the MHC make-up of the child. It denies the right of the child to be vaccinated and so be protected against serious illness and possible death.

Finally, is it possible to predict whether a person will be at great risk of serious disease from certain infections? The answer is—not quite yet. The most effective way would be to analyse all the class I and II T cell epitopes in the proteins of infectious agents, and determine which MHC proteins they bind to with high affinity. Then to analyse the specificity of the MHC proteins, i.e., the HLA haplotype (Table 4.3) of individuals, to see whether they contain the most effective alleles (corresponding to MHC protein specificities) for the different diseases. This approach has already started. Generally, it has been rather harder to make effective vaccines against bacteria than against viruses. To facilitate anti-bacterial vaccine development, the complete DNA sequence of the genomes of about ten important bacteria, including *M. tuberculosis* had been determined by about mid-1998, and about another 15 analyses were then underway (Moxon, 1998). This will provide a catalogue of the genes coding for factors such as those causing serious disease (the virulence of the organism), for promising protein candidates as targets for neutralising antibody production as well as potential T cell epitopes for binding to common class I and II major histocompatibility complex (MHC) proteins in different populations. This approach is already paying dividends as is described in Chapter 9, by the discovery of a gene coding for a protein called Dam, which is necessary for salmonella strains to cause disease in mice.

A simpler but less definitive approach is to divide people suffering from a particular infection into two groups—those who suffer little if any clinical disease, and those who have serious disease. In this way, it is possible to see whether the possession of particular MHC protein specificities is associated with resistance or susceptibility to a particular infectious disease. Some associations of this type have been found with HIV, with malaria and more recently with chlamydia infections. The influence of these findings on recent approaches to vaccine development to these infectious agents is discussed in Chapter 10.

In this chapter, examples of major epidemics of childhood infections and the very rapid effect of mass immunisation in reducing disease incidence have been described. The data provided by the US Centers of Disease Control and Prevention show the extraordinary effectiveness of most of the vaccines against childhood infections. In contrast, in 1994 in the USA and elsewhere, there were still high levels of sickness and considerable mortality due to two other readily transmitted childhood infections, rotavirus and respiratory syncytial virus, for which vaccines were not then available. Finally, because an individual's T lymphocyte response is determined by their particular genetic make-up, individuals will vary in their resistance and susceptibility to different infections. In principle, vaccination is an especially important safety procedure to protect against serious illness (and possible death) if an individual is genetically particularly susceptible to an infection. Because determining resistance or susceptibility to different infectious diseases is not yet feasible on a large scale, it is much better to 'play safe' and be vaccinated wherever possible.

6

Vaccine safety

No vaccines are without some adverse effects. Indeed, there are no medicines, whether synthetic compounds or so-called natural medicines, such as herbal preparations from plants, which do not cause side effects or adverse reactions in at least some individuals on some occasions. Vaccines are no different from other medicines in this respect. Health care workers have often played down the likelihood that immunisation will cause adverse reactions, because of a genuine belief that the diseases themselves are hundreds to thousands times more dangerous than the side effects. As discussed in Chapter 8, 'Addressing parental concerns', when diseases are common, permanent damage (for example, paralysis caused by polio) and death due to complications of the disease are frequent and clearly evident in the community. Consequently, the advantages of immunisation are also clearly evident, and parents need little convincing that the risks of the disease greatly outweigh the risks of vaccines.

As diseases become rare, however, parents may become more concerned about side effects of vaccines. Parents in industrialised countries today have little or no first-hand knowledge of most of the diseases being prevented. Polio and tetanus are diseases of the Third World, as intangible as the risk of being struck by lightning or attacked by a shark when at the beach. The media is likely to fuel parental concerns about immunisation with sensational stories about the dangers of vaccines, often wildly exaggerated, but more likely to sell copy than stories about the disappearance or continued suppression of dangerous infectious diseases.

A schema of the possible timetable of introducing a new vaccine is shown in Figure 6.1. Prior to the introduction of the vaccine, there is a series of epidemics with possibly frequent explosive outbreaks of disease (see the data for measles in the USA, Figure 5.2, as an example). Once the vaccine is introduced, the incidence of disease falls often precipitously (see Figure 5.2 for measles; Figure 5.3 for Hib; and Figure 5.1 for pertussis (whooping cough)). Provided the level of vaccination coverage remains high, the incidence of disease remains low, and the data for several childhood diseases in the USA shows this very clearly (Table 5.1). The introduction of *H. influenzae* type b (Hib) vaccines in the USA, Europe and Australia in the 1990s led within three years to a rapid and sustained fall in cases of meningitis and other infections such as pneumonia caused by Hib. Should an event occur which seriously interrupts

Figure 6.1   Theoretical timetable of vaccine uptake and disease rates after introduction of a new vaccine, and the likely recurrence of disease if vaccine uptake subsequently declines

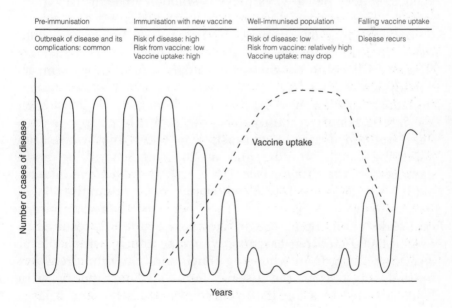

Pre-immunisation	Immunisation with new vaccine	Well-immunised population	Falling vaccine uptake
Outbreak of disease and its complications: common	Risk of disease: high Risk from vaccine: low Vaccine uptake: high	Risk of disease: low Risk from vaccine: relatively high Vaccine uptake: may drop	Disease recurs

vaccine uptake, then it is certain that the disease will recur, as indicated on the right hand side of Figure 6.1. This has been seen in recent years when vaccine delivery was interrupted in some countries in the former USSR. But the classic case was with the pertussis vaccine during the 1970s in the UK.

There is variation in the efficacy of vaccines. The Hib vaccine is highly protective for the vast majority (around 98 per cent) of children, so vaccine failures are rare. As a result, only 2 per cent of children will be susceptible (unprotected) despite immunisation, most children are immunised, the organism stops circulating in the community, and the disease rapidly declines in incidence (Figure 5.3).

In contrast, whooping cough vaccines are less protective than Hib vaccines. The protection rate varies from one whooping cough vaccine to another. The least effective whooping cough vaccines may only protect half of all children against being infected during an outbreak, whereas the most effective whooping cough vaccines protect 95 per cent of children exposed to infection. It has been clearly shown that children who catch whooping cough despite being immunised get less severe disease than unimmunised children who become infected. Immunisation against whooping cough reduces the severity of the disease, even if it does not always prevent whooping cough. Nevertheless, a vaccine that does not prevent all cases and whose efficacy declines over time, is a sitting duck for adverse publicity. In Britain in the late 1970s, the media promoted fears that the whooping cough vaccine might cause brain damage. Subsequent studies have cast grave doubts on whether whooping cough vaccine *ever* causes brain damage. If it does, then the rate is almost certainly very low, probably no higher than 3 per million doses. In contrast, 1 in 600 babies who catch whooping cough will die and up to 1 in 50 will be brain damaged *by the disease* (see Table 6.1). However, the adverse publicity caused the rate of whooping cough immunisation in Britain to fall from 85 per cent to 31 per cent. The two resultant outbreaks of whooping cough, shown in Figure 6.2, resulted in over 100,000 children catching whooping cough, with at least 36 babies dying from whooping cough and many hundreds left brain-damaged from the disease. Similar adverse publicity in Japan also led to a decline in immunisation rates, and a large

Table 6.1: **Estimated rates of adverse reactions following diphtheria-tetanus-pertussis immunisation compared with complications of natural whooping cough**

Adverse reaction	Whooping cough disease complication rates/100,000 cases	DTP vaccine adverse reaction rates/100,000 immunisations
Permanent brain damage	600–2,000	0.2–0.6
Encephalopathy/encephalitis*	90–4,000	0.1–3.0
Convulsions	600–8,000	0.3–90
Shock		0.5–30

*   including seizures, focal neurologic signs, coma, and Reye syndrome
Reproduced with permission from A.M. Galaska, B.A. Lauer, R.H. Henderson and J. Keja (1984) Indications and contraindications for vaccines used in the Expanded Programme of Immunization. *Bull. World Health Organization.* 62:357–66.

whooping cough outbreak. The British outbreaks clearly established that whooping cough remains a severe, potentially fatal disease, even in countries with the best modern technology to treat cases. Even some health care professionals, who were themselves previously confused and sceptical about the relative risks of vaccine and disease, now became firmly convinced of the continuing need for whooping cough immunisation and

Figure 6.2   Whooping cough notifications: deaths in England and Wales from 1940 through 1993.

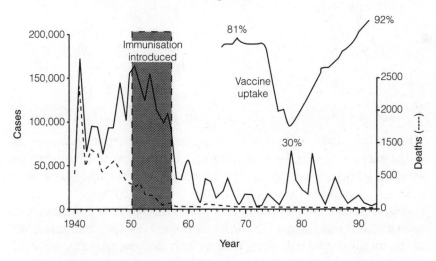

Permission to reproduce this graph in this book was obtained from the Office of National Statistics, 1 Drummond Gate, London

became firm advocates. Immunisation rates subsequently rose and have been maintained at a high level, with over 95 per cent of children being fully immunised. There have been very few cases of whooping cough and no deaths in Britain since immunisation levels improved. The similarity between Figures 6.1 and 6.2 is evident.

ADVERSE EVENTS

Vaccine administration may be associated, over time, with the occurrence of 'adverse events' (adverse reactions). Despite a continuous search for safer and more effective vaccines no vaccine is completely free of side effects, and some adverse events are expected. Fortunately most are relatively mild and self-limiting.

The World Health Organization refers to three types of adverse events:

- programme-related;
- reactions related to the inherent properties of the vaccine; and
- coincidental.

Programme-related

The commonest adverse events caused by programmatic errors are sterile abscesses following inadvertent injection of poorly mixed adsorbed (i.e., mixed with alum) vaccines. Another is lymphadenitis (swollen glands due to infection).

Reactions related to the inherent properties of the vaccine

Adverse events may be due to reactions to different components of the vaccine such as antibiotics (kanamycin or neomycin in measles vaccine, streptomycin or neomycin in oral polio vaccine) or aluminium adjuvant in adsorbed vaccines.

Most such adverse events are relatively mild local reactions (redness and swelling at the injection site) or systemic reactions (fever, rash). Rarely, however, they can be devastating, such as vaccine-associated paralytic poliomyelitis which occurs once in about every 2.5 million doses of the vaccine.

Coincidental

Babies and young children are being immunised at an age when they are often catching viruses and getting infections. It is important to realise that rashes, fevers and other more serious events may be due to concurrent infection, occurring by chance at the same time as the immunisation, and not necessarily caused by the vaccine. The best illustration of this was an elegant study done in Finland by Peltola and Heinonen in 1986. They immunised 581 pairs of twins with the measles-mumps-rubella (MMR) vaccine at one year of age. To sort out which events were due to the MMR vaccine and which were occurring by chance, they gave each twin two injections. For the first injection one twin was given an injection of either MMR or an inactive placebo, while the other twin was given the other injection. Neither the doctor nor the parents knew which twin received MMR and which received placebo. Then, three weeks later, the twin that received MMR was given placebo and the other twin was given MMR, still in a 'blinded' fashion. The parents recorded data on rashes, fever and so on. Only once the data was recorded did they find out whether each twin received MMR on the first or second visit. They were thus able to compare reactions to MMR vaccine and to placebo (i.e. chance). The vast majority of adverse events were equally likely to occur following placebo as following MMR—they were temporally (time) related but not causally related. Fever and/or rash a few days after an injection was more likely to occur after MMR than after placebo. However, respiratory symptoms were no more common after MMR than after placebo, and were very common. MMR vaccine does not cause colds, but children often get colds at the time they are being given MMR vaccine.

THE NATURE OF ADVERSE EVENTS

The severity of adverse events related to immunisation may be perceived differently by the individuals concerned. What is perceived as a mild side effect by a health care professional may be perceived very differently by a worried mother and father. For example, prolonged high-pitched screaming for some hours, resolving without any complications, may be deeply distressing to the child's carers, even if categorised by health workers as 'benign'.

The following adverse events are recognised by health care professionals:

Local reactions

Redness and/or swelling at the injection site is commonest with the triple vaccine (diphtheria-tetanus-whole cell pertussis or DTPw) but also occurs with other vaccines. Local reactions are very common. In a recent Australian study, 70 to 90 per cent of babies had a local reaction to their first, second or third dose of triple vaccine. The rate of local reactions did not increase with subsequent doses, so this was not an allergic reaction. Indeed, local reactions are thought to be due to irritants in the vaccine and not to allergy. The rate of local reactions to DTPw was lower in the United Kingdom, around 10 per cent following the third dose, where DTPw is given at 2, 3 and 4 months, as opposed to 2, 4 and 6 months in Australia. On the other hand, local reactions are much less common, less than 10 per cent, with pertussis vaccines made from purified sub-components of pertussis (acellular pertussis vaccines) compared to whole cell pertussis vaccines.

Fever

Fever following immunisation is common and can cause irritability. Febrile convulsions occur in about 1 in 10,000 one-year-olds immunised with measles vaccine, but these children all recover normally. In contrast, febrile convulsions occur in about 1 in 200 children who catch measles (Table 6.2).

Prolonged crying

Prolonged, often high-pitched, crying persisting for three or more hours is most common in babies after diphtheria-tetanus-pertussis vaccine (triple vaccine). The reason is unclear, but may be related to pain or a sense of insult. It is less common with the new vaccines which incorporate acellular pertussis vaccine, i.e., diphtheria-tetanus-acellular pertussis (DTPa) as opposed to diphtheria-tetanus-whole cell pertussis (DTPw) vaccines.

Table 6.2   Estimated rates of serious adverse reactions following measles immunisation compared with complications of natural measles infection and background rates of illness

Adverse reaction	Measles disease complication rates/100,000 cases	Measles vaccine adverse reaction rates/100,000 immunisations
Encephalitis/encephalopathy	50–400	0.1
Subacute sclerosing panencephalitis	0.5–2.0	0.01–0.1
Pneumonia	3800–7300	Nil
Convulsions	500–1000	0.02–190

Reproduced with permission from A.M. Galaska, B.A. Lauer, R.H. Henderson and J. Keja (1984) Indications and contraindications for vaccines used in the Expanded Programme of Immunization. *Bull. World Health Organization.* 62:357–366.

Hypotonic–hyporesponsive episodes

These so-called HHEs are rare but frightening episodes, occurring 1 to 24 hours after an immunisation, in which the baby goes pale, floppy and unresponsive. They are commoner with DTPw than with DTPa, and commoner with DTPa than with vaccines containing no pertussis components, suggesting pertussis is an important but not the only contributing factor. They occur too late to be classed as faints, although they look like one. Fortunately all children recover fully from HHEs and, once recovered, follow-up studies have shown they return completely to normal. Children who had an HHE after DTPw should be given DTPa for subsequent doses. Interestingly though, when a second dose of DTPw was given to children who had previously experienced an HHE with their first dose, none of the children had a repeat HHE.

Syncope (fainting)

School age children may often faint at the time of or soon after being given an immunisation. They go pale, sweaty and will fall to the ground if not supported. They recover quickly when lain down, but otherwise can hurt themselves by falling. Syncope is another name for a simple faint.

Syncopal fit

Occasionally a fainting child will have a short episode of twitching of the face or limbs. This is known as a syncopal fit or convulsion. They are surprisingly common, and virtually never cause any long-term damage.

Encephalopathy

Encephalopathy is a rather vague term implying an impairment of normal brain function resulting in altered consciousness, such as coma, confusion or convulsions. Children with encephalopathy may recover completely or be left with permanent brain damage. Encephalopathy from any vaccine is extremely rare.

Encephalitis

Encephalitis is a term meaning encephalopathy due to brain inflammation. Like encephalopathy, it is extremely rare. For example, it has been estimated that one in a million doses of measles vaccine causes encephalitis. In contrast about one in a thousand children who catch measles will develop encephalitis from the disease.

Anaphylaxis

Anaphylaxis is an immediate collapse due to an allergic reaction to a vaccine. It is extremely rare, occurring with an incidence of 1 to 3 per million doses of vaccines, which is fortunate as anaphylaxis is potentially life-threatening.

THE TIMING OF ADVERSE EVENTS

Immediate (within 24 hours)

Most (but not all) local and systemic reactions to a vaccine occur within 24 hours of administration of the vaccine, and are caused by inherent properties of the vaccine. It should not be forgotten, however, that events may occur around the time of immunisation by coincidence. For example, in many industrialised countries, immunisations are given to babies at age 2, 4 and 6 months. The peak age of sudden infant death syndrome (SIDS) is 2–6 months. It is easy to suggest that vaccines *cause* SIDS, and this suggestion has been made by many anti-immunisation groups. But, SIDS occurred just as commonly before immunisations were introduced. Indeed, most studies comparing unimmunised and immunised babies show that immunised babies are *less* likely to die from SIDS, in other words that immunisation actually protects against SIDS. This shows the importance of not assuming that, because two events occur at the same time, one caused the other.

Intermediate (1–28 days)

Some adverse events related to a vaccine may occur after a delay of days to weeks. Sometimes there is a logical explanation as to why the adverse event is delayed. For example, measles vaccine is a live, attenuated vaccine, that is, the measles virus is alive although less virulent than wild-type virus. It takes some 7 to 10 days to replicate to its full extent, so that fever and rash occurring 7 to 10 days after measles or MMR vaccine is likely to be caused by the vaccine. Likely to be, but not definitely caused by the vaccine, remembering Peltola's twin study in which fever and rash occurred in babies given placebo but occurred more commonly in babies given MMR.

Mumps vaccine virus replicates even more slowly than measles virus. One mumps vaccine, no longer in use, caused mumps meningitis in a proportion of vaccine recipients, occurring about three weeks after the vaccine was given.

There has been a long-standing debate on whether or not whole-cell pertussis vaccine causes encephalopathy some days after whooping cough immunisation. The problem is that some babies with epilepsy will have their first ever convulsion at age 2–6 months and this will coincide with whooping cough immunisation by chance. This debate started in the medical literature, was taken up by the press and resulted in a fall in pertussis immunisation in the United Kingdom and Japan, with huge outbreaks of whooping cough and many deaths, as outlined above. The risk of encephalopathy caused by the whole cell vaccine was first examined in a British study, the National Childhood Encephalopathy Study, in 1978–81. This study found that one in 100,000 doses of the vaccine caused an encephalopathic illness, but that two-thirds of the affected babies recovered completely. The risk of brain damage due to the vaccine was therefore quoted as 1 in 300,000 doses. This study was based on small numbers of children with encephalopathy, and later follow-up suggested that almost all the children with brain damage 'caused' by the vaccine in fact had underlying brain conditions. These underlying conditions were being uncovered by the vaccine but not caused by the vaccine.

The American Institute of Medicine has examined the evidence as to whether or not whole cell pertussis vaccine causes encephalopathy and/or brain damage. Their conclusion is that the evidence does not permit a clearcut answer. It is possible that whooping cough vaccine does not cause encephalopathy at all. However, if whole cell pertussis vaccine does cause encephalopathy, then their highest estimate of the risk is 1 case in 100,000 doses of the vaccine. It should not be forgotten, however, that for those catching the disease from a whooping cough infection, the risk of encephalitis is much higher (see Table 6.1) than for those immunised with the whole cell vaccine. It is very likely (but unproven) that the risk of this adverse effect following vaccination with acellular pertussis is extremely low.

Long term (over 28 days post-vaccine)

The hardest adverse events to evaluate are those that purportedly occur a considerable time after the immunisation. For example, there has been a recent suggestion of a possible link between measles immunisation and autism. This suggestion was made on the basis of the most tenuous of anecdotal links, without any substantial evidence or any logical scientific explanation as to why there might be a link between measles vaccine and autism but not between measles and autism. However, it is difficult to refute totally such a suggestion. Autism is rare and difficult to define. It occurs in countries which do not give MMR vaccine, but cases are less likely to be diagnosed in such countries. The suggested link between MMR vaccine and autism was not made by anti-immunisation activists, but by medical practitioners in a renowned medical journal. Subsequently, many other experts contributed to the scientific discussion, and it is now considered that MMR does not cause autism. This is an illustration of the kind of difficulties experienced by advocates of immunisation in refuting possible links, such as that between immunisations and AIDS or immunisations and cancer, when there is no rationale to link the two. It has been suggested that immunisation might 'weaken the immune system' and cause problems many years later, but there is no evidence for this. In contrast, some infections such as measles and HIV (AIDS) do weaken the immune system.

Assigning causality

How do we know whether immunisation causes other events that occur at the same time or whether they coincide by chance? In other words, how do we assign causality? The most direct way is to see whether a live agent in the vaccine is directly involved. Thus, the virus isolated from those with paralysis following oral polio vaccine (OPV) administration has been shown to have the properties of the vaccine strain and not of the wild-type strain. This is accepted as scientific proof that the vaccine results in rare cases of paralysis (VAPP). This is the only case where it has been proved scientifically that the vaccine has caused a major disability at such a low incidence.

A more common way, as described above, is to compare the rate that the event occurs in a group of children who are immunised with the rate in an unimmunised 'control' group. This is possible with SIDS because it is a relatively common event (about 1 per 1000 children). However, a large so-called controlled trial is often not practical for rare events. Another approach is to look at the timing of the rare event relative to the date of immunisation. For example, by chance a child may die from SIDS on the same day as they are immunised. This looks and feels to everyone as if the vaccine must have caused the SIDS. But if they occurred on the same day by coincidence, then it would be equally likely for a baby to die from SIDS the day before it was due to be immunised. Studies examining the time of SIDS have shown no increase in the rate of SIDS on the day of or the day after immunisation. So we conclude that if a baby dies from SIDS on the day it was immunised that this is a coincidence. Given that a baby receives a vaccine every 60 days, and assuming that almost all babies with SIDS die at age 2 to 6 months, then on average 1 in every 60 babies that dies from SIDS will die, *by chance*, on the same day it is immunised. That means 1 in 60,000 babies in Australia every year, or roughly four babies a year, will die from SIDS on their immunisation day.

The approach of looking at the timing of rare events in relation to the timing of vaccine is a powerful tool, provided that reporting of these events is accurate and complete. An American study looked at reports of encephalitis in relation to measles vaccine. Cases of encephalitis occurred from the day after measles vaccine as commonly as two weeks later. This probably represents the background rate of encephalitis which occurs irrespective of measles vaccine, and would have been equally likely to occur the day before measles vaccine was given. However, out of the millions of children who received a measles vaccine between 1970 and 1993, 48 developed encephalopathy within the next 14 days. On days 8 and 9 post-measles vaccine, there was a doubling in the number of reports of this syndrome (see Figure 6.3). This suggests that measles vaccine actually *causes* encephalitis after 8 to 9 days, and indeed the timing of replication of measles vaccine virus, a live virus, is consistent with this. To put it in perspective, one in a million or more doses of the measles vaccine virus causes encephalitis, compared with natural measles which causes encephalitis in one in a thousand children—a thousand times more often than

Figure 6.3   Daily onset of encephalopathy after the administration of the first dose of MMR, MR or further attenuated measles vaccine in 48 children between 1970 and 1993.

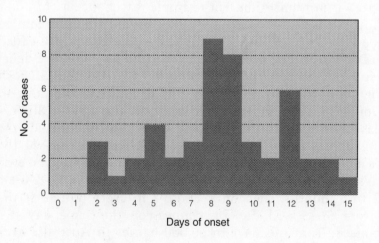

Days of onset

(From *Pediatrics*. 101: 383–7, 1998).
Permission to reproduce this graph was granted by the publishers.

the vaccine. Once linkages between vaccination and a serious adverse effect are proposed, an expert panel may be formed, sometimes by the WHO, to assess the data. Two examples are:

1   An anti-vaccination lobby in France recently claimed that vaccination with the hepatitis B virus vaccine could result in multiple sclerosis (MS). With the assistance of experts in neurology, the WHO subsequently concluded that there was no available scientific evidence to demonstrate a causal association between this vaccination and any central nervous system disease, including MS.

2   It has also been claimed that vaccination with the *Haemophilus influenzae* vaccine (Hib) can lead to the development of diabetes mellitus, an autoimmune disease. In 1998, a workshop to discuss this claim was held at the Johns Hopkins School of Public Health, Baltimore. It concluded 'no vaccines have been shown to increase the risk of type 1 diabetes in humans'. A comprehensive study in Finland found no association between administration of the Hib vaccine and the later incidence of diabetes.

Table 6.3 provides a summary of what is currently known about vaccines and rare events which might be causally or temporally associated.

MONITORING SIDE EFFECTS OF VACCINES

Almost all health care professionals are strong advocates of immunisation. One complaint of the anti-immunisation lobby is that insufficient attention is paid to side effects or adverse events. Such criticism is largely unfounded. In Australia, there is notification of adverse events related to administration of any vaccine. This is co-ordinated on a statewide basis with notification to state representatives as outlined in the NHMRC Immunisation Procedures Handbook published by the Federal Government. In addition, individuals—medical or non-medical—can notify adverse reactions to any vaccine direct to the Adverse Drug Reactions Advisory Committee (ADRAC) in Canberra. During the 1998 campaign to immunise all school children with measles-mumps-rubella (MMR) vaccine, specific surveillance for adverse reactions was instituted as part of the

Table 6.3   Rare conditions and their relationships to vaccines

Rare condition	Vaccine or vaccines	Attributable risk
HIV/AIDS	Any	No evidence that any vaccine causes or predisposes to AIDS. Potential for transmission of AIDS if a needle is used to immunise more than one child, but this is against all recommendations.
Allergy	Any	Good evidence that vaccines do NOT cause allergy.
Asthma	Any	Good evidence that vaccines do NOT cause asthma.
Autism	Measles	Good evidence that measles vaccine does NOT cause autism.
Encephalitis	Measles	Occurs with about 1 in 1,000,000 doses of vaccine (but about 1 in 1,000 cases of natural measles).
Encephalopathy	Pertussis (whole cell)	Risk may be zero or may be as high as 1 in 100,000 doses. Risk thought to be less for acellular vaccine but no good data yet.
Guillain-Barre syndrome (polyneuritis)	Influenza	About 1 in 1,000,000 doses. This estimate is based on epidemiological data
Infantile spasms	Pertussis (whole cell)	Good evidence that pertussis vaccine does NOT cause infantile spasms.
Multiple sclerosis (MS)	Any	No evidence that any vaccine causes MS, but insufficient evidence to totally refute the possibility.
SIDS	Triple vaccine, other vaccines	Good evidence that vaccines do NOT cause SIDS and may even protect against SIDS.
Vaccine-associated paralytic poliomyelitis (VAPP)	Polio vaccine	VAPP occurs once in about every 2,500,000 doses of the live oral polio vaccine. It does not occur with the killed injected polio vaccine.

programme. In addition, Professor Terry Nolan's research group in Melbourne has published a number of studies on the rates of common side effects of vaccines.

In the USA, the Food and Drug Administration maintains continuing surveillance of adverse events after vaccination through its national Vaccine Adverse Event Reporting System (VAERS). This system is a so-called passive surveillance system, relying on health care professionals and vaccine suppliers to notify reports of side effects. As such it has some recognised limitations. Adverse events are under-reported, as is the case with all passive surveillance. There are probable biases, such as how new is the vaccine and the effect of recent publicity about possible adverse events. Events are reported which may not have been caused by the vaccine. VAERS has strengths, too. It is a national reporting system, covering the entire US population. It is a powerful tool for assessing the safety of newly marketed vaccines, and is useful for generating warning signals about possible rare events. For example, in 1998 a study was set up to investigate reports to VAERS about a possible link between influenza vaccine and a rare neurological condition called Guillain-Barre syndrome. This study showed that one in a million doses of influenza vaccine caused Guillain-Barre syndrome in the vaccine recipient. This rare adverse reaction needs to be weighed against the dangers of catching influenza. In one particular situation, the outbreak of 'swine influenza' in 1977–78 in the USA, when about 40 million Americans were immunised, the incidence of Guillain-Barre syndrome was higher, about 1 in 60,000 vaccinations but this high incidence was never seen before this occasion and has not been seen since.

The current status of rare events and their possible relation to vaccines is shown in Table 6.3.

COST OF VACCINE ADVERSE EVENTS

When the costs to the population of a vaccine-preventable disease are compared with the cost of the vaccine, in terms of both vaccine delivery and adverse events, the analysis is almost always in favour of the vaccine and usually by a considerable margin. This is true whether the comparison is of 'human costs', lives saved and handicap prevented, or some sort of estimate of financial costs.

Nevertheless, there are costs involved with vaccine adverse events. For relatively minor adverse events these may be merely the cost of parental anxiety and a visit to the doctor. For severe adverse events, they may be considerable and last the child's lifetime. Who pays? In countries where there is a free health service funded by taxes such as the UK and Australia it has been argued that the child's future care is assured by the welfare state. The USA, on the other hand, has opted for a no fault compensation scheme, funded by a tax on all vaccines. Parents who feel their child has suffered a vaccine-related adverse event apply for compensation. The claim is assessed by an independent panel. Contrary to expectations there has been no shortfall in funds to pay for the compensation claims. The system appears to be 'fair', but in practice the compensation is being paid for by the public in terms of more expensive vaccines. The greatest advantage of the US no fault compensation scheme is that litigation against vaccine companies no longer dominates the equation.

COST OF VACCINES

There are two forms of polio vaccine. Salk vaccine is a killed polio virus, which has to be injected (hence injectable polio vaccine, IPV), while Sabin vaccine is a live oral polio vaccine (OPV). They are both highly and probably equally effective in preventing poliomyelitis. However, OPV is much cheaper to buy and to give and is used in non-industrialised countries, as well as many others including Australia and the United Kingdom. About one in 2.5 million doses of OPV will cause poliomyelitis (vaccine-associated paralytic poliomyelitis, VAPP) in a recipient or a contact of the recipient. The USA now recommends that IPV be given for the first two doses of polio, and OPV thereafter. Australia and the UK have argued that VAPP is sufficiently rare (only one case in Australia in 30 years) and the difference in cost of IPV and OPV is such that the money that would be spent on IPV is better spent on vaccines against other diseases.

Whole cell pertussis vaccine has a chequered history. Some whole cell vaccines are highly effective as in the UK, some as in Canada are poorly protective. Whole cell vaccines are generally very 'reactogenic', with a very high incidence of side effects. In a recent Australian study, 90 per cent of parents reported some sort of adverse event with triple vaccine (DTPw) although almost all were minor and short-lived. Vaccines containing acellular pertussis vaccine (DTPa) cause far fewer minor side effects, but are almost ten times as expensive in Australia. In 1999 in Australia, the government decided to fund DTPa for all immunisations. DTPa is also recommended in the USA. In contrast, the UK continues to use DTPw, arguing that the 2, 3, 4 month schedule results in a low incidence of side effects, that vaccine uptake is over 95 per cent, and that pertussis is extremely rare.

THE MEDIA

The media can play an important role in promoting immunisation, and indeed a recent article by researchers Leask and Chapman found that 95 per cent of Australian newspaper articles were in favour of immunisation. Most of the time, the media are highly responsible on immunisation. On the other hand the media thrive on controversy and sensationalism, and there is considerable potential to do damage, albeit inadvertently, to the public's perception of immunisations and hence to child health.

There can be a dichotomy in perception of the relative hazards associated with vaccines and diseases between industrialised and non-industrialised countries. Vaccine-preventable diseases are rare in the former and common in the latter. An example of this dichotomy was a two-part ABC television programme on immunisation in the Quantum series shown in Australia in 1996. This programme on immunisation was said to give equal time to those who supported immunisation and those who were opposed, but many benefits of vaccination were not presented. The pregnant presenter was trying to decide whether or not to have her child immunised, and at the end of the two-part programme was still undecided. When shown in Australia this programme, in which one of the authors of this book made a brief appearance, caused a storm with immunisation providers and experts in infectious diseases. It is difficult to gauge what effect it had on the public, but a scheduled re-screening of the programme was cancelled, after many complaints that it might cost children's lives if immunisation rates were to fall substantially. Shortly after being shown in Australia, the programme was shown, as are many Australian TV programmes, in Papua New Guinea. In PNG the programme was met with puzzled bewilderment. In a country where the complications of vaccine-preventable diseases are a daily reality, people were astonished that Australians would waste their time agonising over extraordinarily rare side effects of vaccines. To the Papua New Guineans it was equivalent to worrying that an antibiotic might cause a rash or diarrhoea when you were using it to prevent death by a very dangerous infection.

The whooping cough vaccine controversy in the United Kingdom and Japan, already described in some detail, cost a number of lives and left a larger number of children brain damaged. The media raised the level of parental concerns and unwittingly, therefore, might have contributed to the damage of some children's health by denying them the benefits of immunisation. Gangarosa and colleagues in an article in the *Lancet* in 1998, have argued that anti-vaccine movements have at times disrupted pertussis immunisation in Australia, Ireland, Italy, Japan, Sweden, the UK, the former West Germany and Russia. In contrast, in countries without strong anti-vaccine movements, namely the USA, the former East Germany, Hungary and Poland, DTP immunisation levels have remained high, and the incidence of whooping cough is 10 to 100 times lower than in the countries with anti-vaccine movements. Some elements of the press, by publicising anti-vaccine movements, may be partly instrumental in this unfortunate increase in whooping cough and thus in causing deaths and disability. The public clearly has a right and a need to know about both the benefits and the risks of immunisation. Achieving a balance between information and sensationalism is sometimes difficult, but of great importance.

RISKS AND BENEFITS

The risks of serious adverse events following administrations of vaccines are extremely low. This is true whether or not the vaccine-preventable disease is common or rare. Almost all serious adverse events caused by the vaccine can also be caused by the disease, and usually hundreds to thousands of times more frequently (see Tables 6.1 and 6.2). If the disease is now rare, however, a parent may feel that the risk of the vaccine outweighs the risk of the disease. If many parents feel this way, immunisation rates decline, and the disease recurs, often with a vengeance as with diphtheria in the Confederation of Independent States (Russia) in the 1990s or whooping cough in the UK and Japan in the 1970s and 1980s.

The relative risks and benefits of vaccines then are not static. When the disease is common, the benefits of vaccines are obvious. When the disease has become rare as a result of mass immunisation, the risks of vaccines appear greater. This may be an illusion, since if immunisation is withheld from a number of children the benefits of herd immunity are lost and the risks of disease recur.

Vaccines, like other medications, cause side effects. Most side effects are relatively mild, although they may occur very commonly. It is important that health care professionals do not ignore or play down these risks when talking to parents. Parents need to be fully informed about the risks and benefits of immunisation. They also need to be informed about the risks of vaccine-preventable diseases, and the risks of epidemics if children are not vaccinated. Surveillance for both common and rare side effects of vaccines is important to identify new or rare problems, just as is done for other medicines.

7

The crowning achievement— the eradication/ elimination of some human infectious diseases

The concept of 'eradication' of an infectious disease was first used by veterinarians in the United States when they managed to rid that country of diseases of livestock that had been imported from other continents, for example, bovine contagious pneumonia (eradicated 1889) and subsequently foot-and-mouth disease. In the second half of the twentieth century, outbreaks of infection of chickens with virulent forms of influenza (commonly called fowl plague) were contained by the slaughtering of large infected flocks. Such campaigns succeeded because they were able to use quarantine and slaughter as a method of control. This was clearly not applicable to diseases of humans. In addition, the continuous movement of people from country to country made it essential to consider global eradication as the goal, although nationwide eradication (often called elimination to distinguish it from the global goal) was usually an important first step. For many years, quarantine was used to minimise the danger of entry of infectious diseases into a country. Even now, the possession of a valid vaccination certificate may be required as a condition of entry into some countries.

There were initially some unsuccessful attempts in the Americas to eradicate disease or disease-causing agents—hookworm from 1909, yellow fever from 1915 and the mosquito *Aedes aegypti* from 1934. Then there was a successful campaign to eradicate the recently arrived mosquito *Anopheles gambiae* from Brazil in 1938–40. The first Director-General of the World Health Organization (WHO), Dr Brock Chisholm, a Canadian, suggested in 1953 that the WHO should launch a worldwide campaign to eradicate smallpox. Edward Jenner had suggested about 150 years earlier that the widespread use of cowpox could result in the eradication of smallpox. In the intervening period, improved production methods for the vaccine had come into use and great progress had been made in reducing the level of infections in developed countries by vaccination. This was the first campaign which would depend upon vaccination as its prime tool. The proposal was turned down by the World Health Assembly as being too large and complicated. Yet two years later, the Assembly approved a program to eradicate malaria, a much more difficult and complex problem. Members of the Assembly were mesmerised by the early success of DDT for mosquito control, and the strategy was based on this. The incidence of malaria was reduced in many countries and eliminated on some islands. But resistance to DDT was known to occur even when the campaign was launched and was ultimately to cause it to be abandoned. It was said that the campaign succeeded in eliminating malariologists (because of the focus on one chemical) rather than malaria.

THE GLOBAL ERADICATION OF SMALLPOX, 1966–77

After the defeat of the first proposal in 1953, smallpox was again proposed for global eradication in 1958, on this occasion by the USSR which that year had taken its seat on the Assembly after an absence of several years. The proposed strategy was one that had been successful in their vast country. This involved vaccination of at least 80 per cent of the population in all countries where the disease was endemic, using the recently available freeze-dried vaccine which was much more heat stable. This time, the Assembly approved.

Smallpox fulfilled most of the required criteria for a disease that could be globally eradicated. Three most important factors were:

1 The infection was limited to humans; there was no animal reservoir.
2 There was only one strain of virus and it had constant antigenic properties.
3 Based on many years of experience, a very effective vaccine was available. Although the vaccines available at the time induced a higher than desirable level of adverse reactions, the effects of the disease itself were very much worse.

In the next half-decade, there was steady progress in eliminating the disease in developed countries, but this WHO decision which was based on voluntary compliance, had little impact in many developing countries where the disease remained unchecked. By 1966, there were up to 15 million cases of smallpox and 2 million deaths from the infection per year in 33 endemic countries. By the narrowest of margins, the 19th World Health Assembly voted to allocate special funds for an Intensified Special Eradication Programme. The reason for the close vote was the disappointing experience with the malaria campaign and the general realisation that total eradication of an infectious disease was a particularly daunting task. Some eminent scientists were doubtful about the possibility of success.

D. A. Henderson, from the Centers for Disease Control in Atlanta, was appointed to lead the campaign. Ten years were allotted by the WHO to achieve a precise goal—one previously never set or achieved in the history of international preventive medicine. In October 1977, the last case of endemic smallpox was located in Somalia and treated. (The last person to die of smallpox was a very unfortunate woman who was accidentally infected with smallpox virus which 'escaped' from a laboratory in the UK in 1978).

It was a very busy ten years. Strict requirements for vaccine manufacture to a high standard had to be established and constantly monitored, especially in manufacturing facilities in developing countries. The demand for vaccine became so great that a new method for inoculation into the skin, the use of the bifurcated needle, which was much more economical in vaccine use (see Chapter 4) had to be devised. One of the benefits of this technology was that after a group of people, say in a village, had been vaccinated, a return trip to the group a few weeks later allowed a quick examination to check for the presence on the arm of a scar at the site of inoculation. If present, this demonstrated that the vaccination had been successful. Also very fortunately, smallpox infection rarely resulted in subclinical infection or carrier cases. Generally, vaccination gave good protection against infection by the smallpox virus.

The WHO established an advisory committee to help with a wide variety of problems as they arose, and Frank Fenner, Head of the Department of Microbiology at the John Curtin School of Medical Research, Australian National University, and a recognised expert on pox viruses, became a member. He played a critical role. At one stage during the campaign, there was a report that the smallpox virus had been isolated from a non-human source. After painstaking examination of the data, Fenner showed that the claim was faulty—the finding was a laboratory artefact. Had the claim proved to be correct, the goal of eradication would have been impossible to achieve.

The disease disappeared from individual countries or regions, one by one, and each time a special committee was established to verify the correctness of the claim for disease elimination over a several year period. Fortunately, smallpox was not as easily transmitted as measles. Initially, mass vaccination procedures were followed, aiming for an 80 per cent coverage of a population, but this was expensive and not always reliable. In a country like Bangladesh where the population density was very high, a higher coverage rate was required. As increasing progress was made in reducing the incidence of the disease, a new technology was adopted—case-finding and ring vaccination. Groups of health workers would settle in advantageous locations and wait until a report of an infected person or persons came in from the surrounding area. The health workers would then quickly isolate the infected person(s) and immunise all who had contact with him or her.

Figure 7.1 The parchment certifying the global eradication of smallpox, 9 December 1979.

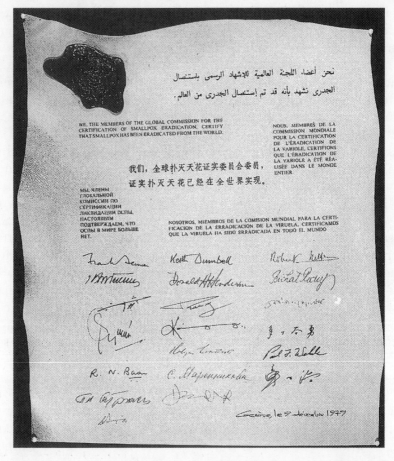

The statement, in five different languages, reads: 'We, the members of the Global Commission for the Certification of Smallpox Eradication, certify that smallpox has been eradicated from the World'.

Permission to reproduce this photograph courtesy of the World Health Organization, Geneva.

There were difficulties of a different kind. In West Africa, there were 23 changes of governments in the participating countries and a major civil war in Nigeria. Ethiopia and Somalia were at war. In August 1976, there was an epidemic in Mogadishu, the capital of Somalia, with over 3,000 cases. It was not resolved until October, 1977. The last case of endemic smallpox globally occurred in Somalia that year.

Figure 7.2   The cover of the World Health Organization magazine of May 1980, declaring that 'smallpox is dead!'

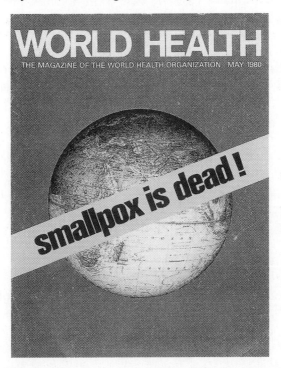

Permission to reproduce this cover, courtesy of the World Health Organization, Geneva.

In 1976, as success of the campaign seemed assured, D. A. Henderson accepted a senior university position in the USA and Isao Arita took over his position as Campaign Director at the WHO. In 1977, Frank Fenner was appointed Chairman of the Global Commission for the Eradication of Smallpox. Its charter was to confirm that global eradication of smallpox had been achieved. In the next three years, there were more than 100 reports of cases of smallpox, a not surprising figure as a substantial financial reward was offered if a positive case was reported. All were investigated and shown to be incorrect (many proved to be chickenpox). In 1980, Frank Fenner reported officially to the World Health Assembly that global eradication of smallpox had been achieved (Figure 7.1). His report was accepted with acclamation and widely publicised (Figure 7.2).

As a result, vaccination of the general public with the smallpox vaccine was stopped in all countries, and has not resumed since.

With Frank Fenner as senior author, the book *Smallpox and its Eradication*—containing over 1400 pages of text and begun in 1980—was published by the WHO in 1988. To honour the overall achievement of smallpox eradication, Henderson, Arita and Fenner shared the Japan Prize in 1988—a recognition of excellence in achievement second only in international status to the award of the Nobel Prize.

There are some people in the groups opposed to vaccination who refuse to believe that smallpox has been eradicated. They may be confusing it with another disease called monkeypox which can infect humans, but cases of human infections by monkeypox virus are relatively rare and confined to Africa. Sequencing of the viral DNA shows conclusively that monkeypox is not the same virus as smallpox. Apparently, however, many of the people opposed to vaccination just do not want to believe that the disease has been eradicated in this way. They do not seem to realise that with the cessation of universal smallpox vaccination in 1980, the smallpox virus, if it was still loose in the world, would be killing millions of people each year.

SMALLPOX IS DEAD! THE MULTIPLE BENEFITS ACCRUING FROM THE GLOBAL ERADICATION OF SMALLPOX

The immediate benefit from the success of the campaign was the prevention each year of two million deaths, several hundred thousand cases of blindness and 10–15 million cases of disease (Figure 7.3). Above all, it was the saving of an enormous amount of human suffering due to this terrible disease.

Some US$1–2 billion in costs of services such as vaccination and treatment of the sick throughout the world, have been saved each year since 1980. The cost to the WHO for the eradication campaign is estimated to have been about US $300 million. In contrast, to put a man on the moon is said to have cost $24 billion! (Both were fantastic achievements.)

In the longer term, an important benefit to humankind is the demonstration that in favorable circumstances, *it is possible* to eradicate a deadly infectious disease. The example of small-

Figure 7.3   Some effects of smallpox infection.

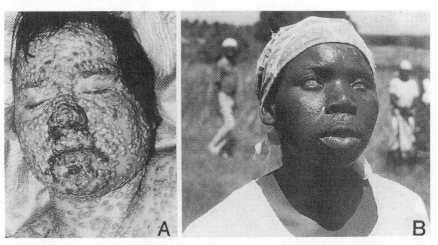

A.   Facial lesions in a severe case of ordinary-type smallpox (later fatal) at the height of the illness.

B.   Blindness could occur following infection, as in this case from Zaire.

Permission to reproduce these photographs courtesy of the World Health Organization, Geneva.

pox has set a precedent for other diseases. It is doubtful that any other eradication programme would have been initiated after 1980 if the smallpox campaign had not been successful because technically, of all the infectious diseases, smallpox offered the best opportunity.

Programmes to eradicate two other virus diseases were initiated, and these will shortly be described. And the question was asked—are there other infectious diseases of global importance which offer the opportunity to interrupt their life cycle in a simple but effective way? The answer is 'yes' and one example will be described towards the end of the Chapter because the technology used is so delightfully simple, and a wonderful example of what can be achieved.

POLIOMYELITIS AND MEASLES AS TARGETS FOR ERADICATION

The two other viral diseases which soon came to be considered as the target for global eradication campaigns were poliomyelitis and measles. Table 7.1 gives a more complete list of factors

Table 7.1   Factors favouring eradication of an infectious disease by vaccination

		Disease		
Factors		*Smallpox*	*Poliomyelitis*	*Measles*
1	Infection is limited to human host	Yes	Yes	Yes
2	Only one or a few strains of virus (Not subject to high rates of mutation)	Yes	Yes	Yes
3	A safe effective vaccine is available	Yes	Yes	Yes
4	The vaccine is heat stable	Yes	No	No
5	Absence of subclinical/carrier cases	Yes	No	Yes
6	Virus is only moderately infectious	Yes	Higher	Highly
7	Ready marker of successful vaccination	Yes	No	No

favouring eradication of an infectious disease by vaccination and makes comparisons between smallpox, polio and measles. They share the three most important characteristics—only a human host, one or a few strains of virus and the availability of a safe and effective vaccine. Importantly, despite the fact that (like influenza) the polio and measles viruses have RNA as their genetic material, they do not show significant changes in antigenic properties although there are three subtypes of polio. In contrast, the viruses differ from smallpox in four respects. Polio causes a high level of subclinical infections, both polio and measles have a higher level of transmissibility and for both there is no easy marker of successful vaccination. To make the task still more challenging, both the polio and measles vaccines are heat labile (affected by heat), so that they must be kept refrigerated until administered—quite a task especially in developing countries in the tropics.

PROGRESS TOWARDS THE ERADICATION OF
    POLIOMYELITIS

In 1985, the Director of the Pan American Health Organization (PAHO, the regional office of the WHO) proposed the initiative to eliminate the indigenous transmission of wild-type polio virus from the whole of the American continent (north and south) by the year 1990. Ciro de Quadros was appointed officer in charge and much of the progress made so far is a tribute to his leadership. The goal set by PAHO was extended in 1988 by the World Health Assembly to achieve global eradication by the year 2000.

Polioviruses are generally transmitted by the faecal–oral route. (The faeces of those infected with polio contains infectious virus which can easily be transmitted by hand to the mouth of another child.) The major site of viral growth is the gut where virus may persist for some weeks. A short-lived viraemia can follow, leading to infection of cells in lymphoid tissues and in the nervous system, and can lead to a paralytic state (acute flaccid paralysis). Two vaccines were available. Use of the inactivated whole virus vaccine (IPV) would prevent the viraemia and hence paralysis. The live attenuated viral vaccine (OPV) results in occasional cases of paralysis due to reversion of the attenuated virus to virulence (1 case per several million doses). Nevertheless, OPV was chosen for use because of its high efficacy, easy administration (oral) and very low cost.

Technically, the difficulties facing an eradication programme were substantial. The OPV vaccine is heat labile, multiple administrations were required, most infections are subclinical (no apparent disease) and there is the need to distinguish between endemic and vaccine-caused or derived paralysis. Also, there is no simple marker (like a scar on the arm) of successful vaccination.

These obstacles were largely overcome by the adoption of four major strategies (Table 7.2). Two of these were especially important in the PAHO initiative—the holding of national immunisation days (NIDs), catch-up and follow-up campaigns so that whole populations were reached, and the establishment of nearly 15,000 health facilities throughout the Americas to report regularly on the presence or absence of cases of paralysis. The last case of indigenous poliomyelitis occurred in Peru in August 1991, and elimination of indigenous cases of this disease in the whole region was declared three years later. This achievement has only been broken by the introduction of infectious cases from outside the Americas, such as by individuals who were unvaccinated because of particular religious beliefs.

This achievement stimulated greater international efforts. In 1988, the WHO Western Pacific region adopted a resolution to eliminate this disease from the region by 1995. After holding several NIDs, China reached this goal just in time, but has to

Table 7.2   WHO strategies for poliomyelitis eradication

1	Achieving and maintaining high routine vaccination coverage among children with at least three doses of oral polio vaccine (OPV);
2	Administering additional doses of OPV to all young children during National Immunisation Days (NIDS) to rapidly interrupt poliovirus transmission;
3	Establishing sensitive systems of routine detection for virus-induced paralysis, and for subsequent isolation of the virus; and
4	Conducting 'mopping-up' vaccination activities, catch-up and follow-up campaigns, i.e., localised campaigns targeted at high-risk areas where poliovirus transmission is most likely to persist or be introduced.

screen cases of paralysis imported from neighbouring countries like Myanmar (Burma). After a tremendous effort in Cambodia, Laos and Vietnam to make sure that every child aged under five years was immunised, the last case of paralytic polio was detected in March 1997 in Cambodia. Australia has been free of indigenous poliomyelitis for some years.

Two particular stories indicate the enthusiastic support for this programme. On one day in December 1997 in India, 123 million young children were vaccinated with OPV by volunteer health workers. The volunteers used almost every conceivable form of transport to reach the children! In countries such as Angola and Afghanistan where civil wars have been raging for as long as 30 years, it was arranged that hostilities cease for one day so that a NID could be held!

The programme has been difficult to implement in three areas: the countries which border the European and eastern Mediterranean regions of the WHO, notably Iraq, Iran, Syria and Turkey; Bangladesh; and Africa. In 1993, the WHO regional task force in Africa called for 41 countries in the region to conduct two NIDs each year for three years. By the end of 1997, 17 countries had reached this goal. As part of the overall plan, Nelson Mandela chaired a committee with the slogan—*Kick polio out of Africa.* There remain substantial difficulties in those countries where major conflicts are in progress, such as Zaire, the Democratic Republic of the Congo and Nigeria. As of May 1999, 6,227 poliomyelitis cases with onset during 1998 were reported, a remarkable achievement. It currently seems unlikely that elimination of polio from some parts of Africa will be achieved by the end of the year 2000.

Figure 7.4 **Children paralysed by poliomyelitis being sustained in iron lungs in the Hall Ward of the Royal Alexandra Hospital for Children in Camperdown, Sydney, during an outbreak in 1937–38. The first poliovirus vaccine (Salk) became available in the early 1950s.**

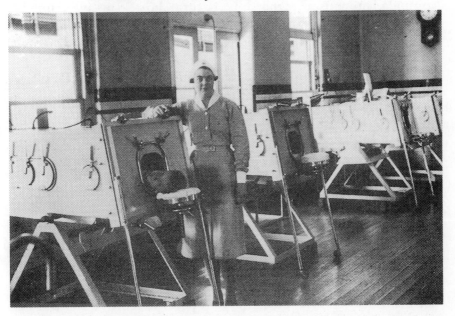

Reproduced with permission of the Royal Alexandra Hospital for Children.

For the poliomyelitis eradication programme to succeed, the momentum must be maintained and even increased. Furthermore, complete vaccination coverage must be continued internationally until eradication is officially declared. Those in charge of the programme realise that if success can be achieved, the experience obtained will greatly enhance the prospects for a successful measles eradication programme because measles is regarded in Africa as a more serious disease than poliomyelitis.

In the late 1940s/early 1950s, there were epidemics of poliomyelitis in a number of countries, including the USA and Australia (Table 5.2). Figure 7.4 shows what was then a common sight—children with permanently paralysed breathing muscles living in iron lungs. Let us hope that very early in the new millennium, we will know that this is a sight which will never be seen again.

CAN MEASLES BE ERADICATED?

Although some subhuman primates can be infected with measles and the virus can be adapted to grow in several laboratory animals, humans are the only natural host. The infection is spread by droplets from the infected respiratory tract; secretions which may be inhaled by others. The virus initially replicates in cells of the upper respiratory tract or in conjunctival epithelium (eyes) after which cycles of viraemia occur so that the virus is distributed around the body, resulting in serious disease. A vaccine composed of a live, attenuated strain has been used very successfully in the WHO Expanded Programme on Immunization. Natural measles infection usually results in lifelong immunity; immunity following vaccination is not so long-lived.

There is evidence that measles transmission can be interrupted by vaccination. This had been achieved in the Gambia (1967–70, until funds ran out), in English Caribbean Islands (1992–), in Cuba and Chile (1993–) and in Finland (1994), using a two-dose schedule.

The goal of measles eradication posed some new challenges for health experts. Whereas the oral polio vaccine (OPV) can be given at birth, the measles vaccine which is administered by injection, will not take in the presence of maternal antibody. In an endemic region, all infants receive specific antibody from their mothers, and this persists for six to nine months. To make sure it will take, the vaccine is given at nine months which means that for those infants whose level of antibody has waned before nine months, there is the strong chance they will be infected before they are vaccinated. This is considered to be the reason for about one million infant deaths due to measles infection each year in endemic countries. Attempts to overcome the problem by using a 'stronger' (high-titre) virus vaccine were stopped because of some deaths which may have been due to the vaccine.

There were potential solutions. One was to develop an entirely new vaccine—one that would be effective at birth in the presence of antibody—but it takes a long time to develop and adequately test a new vaccine. There was an alternative approach. In non-endemic countries, the vaccine is administered between 12 and 18 months as exposure of an infant to the infection is unlikely to occur before then. By following the strategies similar to those devised for the polio campaign— National Immunisation Days (NIDs), catch-up campaigns and follow-up campaigns (Table 7.2), the aim was in effect to convert endemic regions into non-endemic regions over a period of some years.

The second difficulty was the very high transmission rate of the measles virus and the knowledge that all immunisation campaigns would need to obain a coverage of close to 95 per cent. This compared to a figure of about 80 per cent for smallpox.

In 1994, the Pan American Health Organization (PAHO) established the goal of measles elimination in the Americas by the year 2000. In Europe and the Eastern Mediterranean regions, the dates chosen by WHO Regional Centres are 2007 and 2010 respectively. Between 1987 and 1994, more than 136 million children in 15 countries in the Americas (excluding the USA and Canada) had been immunised, a coverage rate of 93 per cent. The rate in the Western Pacific region (including Australia) was also 93 per cent. The overall rates in other regions, especially Africa, are much lower. Despite the encouraging figure for the Americas, there have been measles epidemics there in recent years. The largest was an outbreak in 1997 in the state of São Paulo in Brazil, the one state in that country which did not fulfil the recommended series of immunisations. The epidemic spread to other states in Brazil and neighbouring countries.

Based on the accomplishments with poliomyelitis elimination, it seems likely that elimination of indigenous measles will be achieved in the Americas and in some other regions in due course. For regions like Africa, much will depend upon the outcome of the poliomyelitis eradication campaign.

Measles causes an estimated two million deaths per year globally. It can cause a terrible brain disease—subacute sclerosing panencephalitis or SSPE. Though measles is not dreaded as much as smallpox, it would still be a wonderful achievement if it could be eradicated. PAHO has recently published a measles eradication field guide to facilitate the campaign.

OTHER POSSIBLE CANDIDATES FOR GLOBAL ERADICATION BY MASS VACCINATION

This is a frequent topic for discussion at meetings on infectious diseases. As yet there seems to be no general consensus about the next most likely candidate(s), but mumps and rubella may well be near the top of the list when agreement is reached.

It should be mentioned in passing that there are a number of other infectious diseases where spectacular headway is being made towards global 'containment' so that the disease becomes only a minor public health problem. This is being achieved by using multidrug therapy. The progress being made with one disease in particular, leprosy, is very encouraging. But there is another disease, dracunculiasis, where, by using a very simple public health procedure, global eradication—not just containment—seems quite possible.

THE CASE OF THE GUINEA WORM

We briefly met the guinea worm, a nematode, in Chapter 1. In endemic areas, people drink water containing a minute crustacean (cyclops) that is infected with the nematode larvae, and so acts as a vector. The larvae are liberated in a person's stomach or duodenum from where they migrate through the mucosa, become adults and the female, after mating, migrates to the subcutaneous tisssues, grows and causes the disease. A person with a guinea worm emerging, for example, from the leg, can contaminate one or more water sources and cause an epidemic of dracunculosis one year later. To prevent infection, water can be boiled or chemically treated before drinking, but because of the constant size of the crustacean vector, a simpler approach has been to pass all water for drinking through a filter with a mesh size of 100 microns (a micron is one thousandth of a millimetre). If all humans fail to become infected, it would break the cycle of infection with the crustacean.

A global campaign to eradicate dracunculiasis began in 1980 when scientists from the Centers for Disease Control and Prevention (CDC, Atlanta, USA) began persuading supporters of the International Drinking Water Supply and Sanitation Decade (1981–91) to target this disease for eradication. The (Jimmy)

Carter Center's Global 2000 Program (Atlanta, USA) joined the battle in 1986 and initiated a co-operative programme with Pakistan to eradicate the disease in that country. Eight years later, Pakistan reported zero cases for a full calendar year. The World Summit for Children set the aim of eradicating the disease globally by the year 2000, and a World Health Assembly resolution in 1991 expressed commitment to this goal. By early 1996, it was reported that eradication had been 97 per cent achieved. In 1997–8, Pakistan, Iran, Cuba and Egypt were certified free of dracunculiasis transmission and eight other countries reported very few cases. Sudan had the highest number of cases (43,596) at the end of 1997, due to the continuing racial conflicts there.

When the time arrives, eradication will be declared by a special commission established for this purpose, but declared only if, after extensive investigation over a period of three years, no person in a previous endemic region is found to be infected. Then, filtration of drinking water can cease in those countries where the disease was previously endemic.

Many would regard the eradication of smallpox, a prime candidate for the prize of the most unpleasant of all human infectious diseases, as the greatest achievement in the history of public health. In the long run, a very great benefit from this achievement is the knowledge that in appropriate circumstances, this experience can be repeated. It requires certain commitments in order to succeed. The first is the political determination on the part of the countries to provide the bulk of the infrastructure and the basic support necessary to perform the nominated work in the approved programme. The second requirement for a global effort is the provision of the necessary funds to carry out a programme. These almost invariably come from donors which are usually governments or non-governmental organisations in developed countries. A third requirement is sustainability of effort, particularly on the part of the donors. 'Donor fatigue' can easily set in and scarce funds be diverted to another worthy effort. Fourth, the continuing supply of critical reagents of adequate quality, such as the vaccine, must be guaranteed. Finally, those who initiated the eradication programmes must not waver from their original belief that eradication of poliomyelitis, measles and the guinea worm is absolutely worthwhile.

If these programmes are successful, it is very likely that others will be commenced in the new millennium.

8

Addressing parental concerns

This chapter addresses parental concerns about vaccines and immunisation and attempts to analyse the reasons why some parents either delay or do not get their children immunised.

By far the majority of parents in Australia and other developed countries are pro-immunisation. In a recent survey of three-year-old Melbourne children conducted by Lyndal Bond, Terry Nolan and colleagues, 85 per cent were *completely immunised* and nearly 15 per cent had some but not all their immunisations, and thus were *incompletely immunised*. Only 1 in 200 children had received *no immunisations*. The national figure for children who receive no vaccines is about 1 per cent or 1 in 100 children. This chapter draws heavily on the work of Dr Bond and Associate Professor Nolan, who have kindly agreed for their work to be presented.

WHY DO PARENTS GET THEIR CHILDREN IMMUNISED?

Parents who completely immunise their children perceive vaccine-preventable diseases as being serious, and vaccines as being effective and safe with few serious side effects. They trust their health care provider. Incomplete immunisers tend to perceive vaccine-preventable diseases as being most severe in adults, and feel that young children should either be immunised or get the disease when they are young. These are not valid alternatives. Ironically, most vaccine-preventable diseases, such as whooping cough and measles, are in fact *more* severe in younger children.

Most parents understand the concept of herd immunity; that getting their child immunised not only protects their own child as an individual, but contributes to the immunity of the population and keeps diseases at bay. Thus immunising one's child is seen as a *social responsibility* as well as a responsibility to the child's health and welfare. In Australia and the United Kingdom there is social pressure to immunise children but no statutory requirement. In many other countries there is legislation to make immunisations effectively mandatory. In China over 99 per cent of children are immunised without resort to legislation.

CONCERNS ABOUT IMMUNISATION

The vast majority of the Australian population, around 85–90 per cent, are strongly in favour of immunisation and have few worries about immunisation. A very small minority, 0.5 per cent to 1 per cent, are completely opposed to immunisation. The remaining 10–15 per cent start immunising their children but may delay starting or have trouble completing their child's immunisations (see Table 8.1). The reasons for not completing immunisations are usually technical rather than philosophical. The child keeps getting bad colds just as the next vaccine is due. The child's brothers and sisters get sick. The appointment gets forgotten or something else comes up.

But many people will voice some concerns, and these may contribute to delayed immunisation by raising parental doubts about the importance of immunisation. These concerns are discussed below, and some questions and answers about immunisation are given at the end of this chapter in Table 8.2.

DO VACCINES OVERLOAD THE IMMUNE SYSTEM?

It is commonly felt by parents that giving vaccines, particularly to very young children, may be beyond the capacity of their immune system. There is virtually no evidence to support this suggestion. Babies need to be able to respond immunologically to foreign organisms from birth. Within hours of birth a baby's

Table 8.1   Parental perceptions and immunisation status

Immunisation status	Perception of severity of vaccine-preventable disease	Perception of benefits of vaccines	Barriers to immunisation
Complete (85% of Australians)	Serious	Vaccines safe and effective. Serious side-effects rare	Need trusted health care provider
Incomplete (14.5%)	Best to get vaccine or disease when young. Diseases more serious for adults	Vaccines safe but not very effective. Vaccines reduce severity of disease	Minor illnesses in child or sibling, forget, receive confusing advice, difficult access
None (0.5%)	Not serious	Vaccines dangerous and ineffective	Immunisations seen as 'conspiracy'

Table adapted from Bond, L. (1999).

nose, throat, skin and bowel will have become colonised with dozens of organisms, without any harm to the baby. If the baby's immune system could not cope with these organisms, then the baby would become ill with infection and perhaps die, in practice a rare event. Babies' immunity may not be as good as adults' but it is still excellent. They can respond to some vaccines at birth, such as polio vaccine, hepatitis B vaccine and the BCG vaccine against tuberculosis, and by two months can respond to vaccines containing a number of different organisms. Currently in Australia, the UK, the USA and most other developed countries at two months of age we give babies five different organisms at once, the oral polio vaccine, the diphtheria-tetanus-pertussis vaccine in one syringe and the Hib meningitis vaccine in another syringe. Babies respond well to all five vaccines. We begin as early as two months because of the importance of early protection and because of the good immune response (measured by antibody production and protection against disease). In developing countries, the first DTP vaccine is given even earlier, at six weeks. In future, more vaccines against other organisms are likely to be incorporated and preliminary work has shown that babies will respond to vaccines containing seven or more organisms. The only vaccine that has been shown to suppress the immune system is live measles vaccine. This vaccine causes a brief, transient decrease in immunity. This decreased immunity is much more marked with natural measles infection. The vaccine-induced immuno-suppression is not thought to be clinically significant for normal healthy children. However, one extra strong measles vaccine given to very young babies in developing countries was withdrawn because of concerns about significant immunosup-pression. There is some doubt about whether the post-measles vaccine immunosuppression was true, because the increased mortality from other unrelated infections seen after measles vaccination applied only to girls. The current measles vaccine is not associated with increased susceptibility to other infec-tions, either in developed or developing countries.

The reason that only some but not all vaccines can be given at birth is interesting. Some substances when injected into babies at birth are perceived as 'foreign', and the baby reacts to them by mounting an immune response. Others are perceived as 'self' antigens. The baby not only fails to react to them immunologically when they are injected, but recognises them as self when they are injected again later, and 'tolerates' them by not making a good immune response. This phenomenon is known as tolerance. Vaccines such as diphtheria and tetanus which induce tolerance if given at birth, induce an excellent antibody response if immunisation is delayed until the baby is 6–8 weeks old.

DO VACCINES CAUSE AUTOIMMUNE DISEASE?

Autoimmunity is where the body's immune system reacts against self components. Making antibodies against self proteins and complex sugars is very common despite the special system involving the processing of T lymphocytes in the thymus gland to minimise this effect (see Chapter 4). In most cases, these antibodies do not cause disease. But sometimes disease does occur and there is much research now to try to prevent this (see Chapter 11). Some of these diseases are relatively common, like the different forms of diabetes and arthritis. Can adminis-tration of any vaccine induce autoimmunity or autoimmune disease? It is likely that some vaccines do cause a degree of autoimmunity because of cross-reactivity between antigens in the vaccine with host components. But to date, no convincing evidence has been presented that administration of any vaccine is directly responsible for any later occurrence of a serious autoimmune disease. Two examples where such claims have been investigated are quoted in Chapter 6, under the heading 'Assigning causality'.

TENSION BETWEEN NATURAL OCCURRENCE (DISEASE) AND MEDICAL INTERVENTION (IMMUNISATION)

Jenner's development of the first vaccine against smallpox followed his observation of a completely natural occurrence. Milkmaids, who caught cowpox from cows, had beautiful complexions because they never caught the smallpox. The wholly natural disease cowpox protected against the much more severe (but also 'natural') disease smallpox.

We are not always fortunate enough to have a virus like cowpox to use as a 'natural' vaccine. Consequently live virus vaccines have been employed using the technique of attenuation, in which the virus is grown through multiple generations in controlled conditions until it becomes more benign (less virulent and having less disease-causing potential). Is this unnatural? Well, yes and no. The vaccines are certainly different. They cause much less severe disease, if any at all. The immunity they induce may be quite long-lasting, but is rarely lifelong, so that booster doses are needed. In contrast, some 'natural' diseases like measles confer lifelong immunity, though second attacks of other diseases like whooping cough and rubella (German measles) can occur despite 'natural' immunity.

HOW SERIOUS FOR CHILDREN ARE DISEASES CAUSED BY INFECTIOUS AGENTS?

Perceptions of disease depend on many factors, notably on personal exposure to the disease and its complications, on publicity and on education. Many parents perceive diseases which they see commonly, such as measles, mumps and rubella as being mild in young children, because the great majority of children who catch measles will recover completely. To health care professionals, measles is certainly not mild. In 1990 measles was the eighth commonest cause of death in the world, killing more than lung cancer or road traffic accidents. Most of these deaths were young children in poor countries. But in Australia between 1972 and 1995, measles killed 140 children and young adults, more than all other vaccine-preventable diseases combined. If measles immunisation was stopped in Australia today, there would be 25 deaths a year from measles (due to pneumonia and encephalitis) and more than 30 children each year would be left brain-damaged from measles encephalitis. In contrast, measles vaccine causes one case of encephalitis every four years.

During the debate about whooping cough vaccine, some authorities maintained that whooping cough was no longer a serious disease in industrialised countries. Yet in an outbreak in Australia which lasted 15 months in 1997–98, nine babies died from whooping cough (seven in New South Wales) despite the most modern intensive care.

ILLUSION OF CONTROL

There are situations in which we feel we can control circumstances by our actions, whereas the truth is that some of that control is an illusion. We all recognise that if we are on an aeroplane that crashes, we have little or no control over our fate. When we are driving a car we believe, correctly, that driving sensibly decreases the risk of having an accident. The problem is that we are still at risk from other drivers driving carelessly.

Many parents believe that although disastrous complications of diseases do occur, they will never happen to their child. They particularly believe that if their child is kept healthy by a good diet and regular exercise, then their child is safe.

There is certainly good evidence that malnourished children are at increased risk of severe complications of infectious diseases. The corollary is that healthy children are indeed at lower risk. However, infectious diseases are no respecters of good health, and healthy children *may* suffer severe infections and severe complications, even death. Most children in Australia who died from measles or whooping cough in the last 25 years were previously healthy, well-nourished children. If children don't have a good combination of genes that enable them to develop a strong immune response to a particular infection

(Chapter 5), they can become very sick or die, no matter how healthy they appear to be.

Certainly a healthy lifestyle is good for children, and will improve their ability to fight infections. But suggesting that this is sufficient to protect against all infectious diseases, without the need for immunisation, is like suggesting that you are safe on the roads if you drive carefully, so you do not need seat belts. Infectious diseases are like bad drivers. If you drive well you may still be killed or maimed by a bad driver. A seat belt gives extra protection. Drive safely, but also wear a seat belt. Give your child a healthy lifestyle, but also get them immunised.

THE ANTI-IMMUNISATION LOBBY

Soon after Jenner introduced cowpox vaccination in the 1790s, a cartoon appeared in the satirical journal *Punch* depicting immunised adults turning into cows (Figure 2.3). There is nothing new about anti-immunisation movements. They are usually a small group of well-educated, vociferous individuals. Their knowledge of immunisation may be good, but their interpretation of data differs radically from that of health care professionals. They perceive vaccine-preventable diseases as being mild, not serious, and as being preventable by adopting a healthy lifestyle. All health care professionals are treated with suspicion. Immunisations are painted as being a conspiracy by health care professionals, although since almost all health care professionals immunise their own children, it would be a strange conspiracy in which all children including their own were victims. Anti-immunisation lobbyists may adopt homoeopathic 'immunisation' as an alternative, even though the Royal Homoeopathic Society recommends that homoeopathic 'immunisation' only ever be given *in addition to, but not instead of* conventional medical immunisation.

MAKING DECISIONS ABOUT IMMUNISATION

Omission bias is the term given to the tendency to take no action if that action might cause harm, even if there is a greater risk of harm by doing nothing. Parents may fear getting their child immunised because of the risks of the vaccine, especially when these have been emphasised in the media, and even if intellectually they accept that the disease carries more risks. They will omit the immunisation because they feel *they* are inflicting the risk on the child, rather than let nature take its riskier course. The tragic tale of Benjamin Franklin's son who died from smallpox because his father feared to have him vaccinated, is related in Chapter 2. Frisch and Baron (1988) found that it was not just parents who were vulnerable to omission bias. In their survey of tertiary students without children, 23 per cent of those surveyed thought it was worse to vaccinate a child when the vaccination might harm the child, rather than not vaccinate, even if the vaccine would reduce the *overall* risk of harm.

The way choices are framed is important in decision-making. Tversky and Kahneman framed a study question in which there were two options, say option A and option B, to try to save 600 people at risk. In option A, 200 would certainly be saved but 400 would certainly die. Option B was a 1 in 3 chance of saving all 600. What was fascinating was that people's decision varied greatly on how the problem was framed. If told that option A was a certainty of saving 200 and that option B was a 1 in 3 chance of saving all 600, then 72 per cent of respondents favoured option A. If instead they were told that option A involved a certainty that 400 of 600 would die, whereas option B was a 2 in 3 chance of all 600 dying, then 78 per cent of respondents chose option B.

In other words, if the outcomes of the choice were framed positively, as in the first example, then people would shy away from taking a risk. If the outcomes were framed negatively they were likely to take the risk. There may be a lesson in how health care professionals might talk to parents about immunisation, if immunisation is perceived as the weighing up of the risk of the vaccine against the risk of the disease.

The implication of this research is that parents are more likely to have their children immunised if the risks of immunisation are presented in positive terms rather than negative terms. In other words it might be explained, depending on the degree of detailed information wanted by the parent, that vaccines are almost always safe or there is a 99.999 per cent chance that the child will have no lasting adverse effects of the vaccine. The 'negative' alternative is to say that there is a very small risk of permanent effects from immunisations, perhaps 1 in 100,000 cumulative risk or 1 in 1,000,000 for each vaccine. Of course, it is important to offset these dangers of immunisations against the dangers of *not* immunising, that is, the dangers of the disease.

WHAT DO PARENTS WANT TO KNOW?

Most parents who get their children immunised do so because they trust their health care professionals, they trust the health care system and they believe that immunisations are given for the benefit of their own and other children in the community.

Parents who are uncertain about immunisation feel that health care professionals are not impartial and are very positive about the benefits of immunisation, but woolly about contra-indications. When asked, these parents feel they lack balanced, detailed information and they feel there is poor communication between health care providers and the public. Either the parents who complain of lack of balanced information feel the written information is too partial towards immunisation, or they want more time for detailed verbal discussion with their general practitioner or immunisation nurse.

The Australian Commonwealth Department of Health and Family Services publishes a number of information brochures on immunisation. Some are for parents, such as 'Understanding childhood immunisation'. Others are directed more at health care providers, such as 'Immunisation myths and realities'. These are readily available through State or Federal immunisation and health clinics. Contact phone numbers and addresses are given at the end of this book in Appendix 1.

The data shown in Table 8.1 suggest that partial immunisers are pro-immunisation, but are concerned about vaccine efficacy and are confused about the severity of vaccine-preventable diseases, and which ages are at high risk. They believe that some diseases are not serious for young children. They find structural and service barriers to completing their child's immunisations. One of the main barriers is an identified lack of detailed information and of caring, understanding professionals they feel they can trust. Given that written information in varying levels of detail *is* freely available, either parents are not provided with this information, do not ask for it, or else written information has limited impact and the personal touch of a sympathetic health care professional with time to discuss concerns is what parents really want.

DO VACCINES WORK?

The vaccines used in immunisation programmes are generally highly effective, protecting well over 90 per cent and usually well over 95 per cent of children immunised. These figures mean that 95 in every 100 children exposed to the infection will not become infected if later exposed to the natural infectious agent.

But the situation can vary in different countries and in different circumstances, as is illustrated by the following examples.

Whooping cough

Whooping cough (pertussis) is a highly contagious disease, causing worldwide 20–40 million cases and 200,000 to 400,000 fatalities each year.

Whooping cough vaccines vary in their efficacy. The whole cell whooping cough vaccine used in studies in Sweden and Germany protected over 90 per cent of children against infection, whereas a Canadian whole cell whooping cough vaccine protected less than half of all children immunised. Babies are at highest risk of complications if they catch whooping cough, and whooping cough is one disease where maternal antibody and breast milk do not protect. Babies as young as two weeks can catch whooping cough, often from a sibling or parent with whooping cough. Their best protection is widespread population immunisation, resulting in 'herd immunity'. Currently in the United Kingdom over 95 per cent of babies receive whooping cough vaccine. There is virtually no whooping cough circulating, because of the resultant herd immunity. Babies virtually never catch whooping cough in the UK now because they are never exposed. It is not because UK children are especially healthy.

Before re-unification, in East Germany, where whooping cough immunisation was compulsory, whooping cough was extremely rare. In contrast in West Germany, where only about 11 per cent of children were given whooping cough vaccine, whooping cough still circulated, was severe and killed babies. Yet West Germany was a much richer country than East Germany.

In contrast whooping cough still circulates in Australia because of poor levels of immunisation. Babies are often exposed. The nine deaths from whooping cough in Australia in 1997–98 were all babies too young to have been protected by immunisation, but who were infected by friends and relatives.

The recurrence of outbreaks of severe whooping cough in the UK (in 1977–78) and in Japan, when immunisation levels fell, and the disappearance of these outbreaks when high levels of immunisation resumed (see Figure 6.2), provide compelling evidence that whooping cough immunisation works and that whooping cough is still a devastating disease.

Why then do immunised children still get whooping cough? In Australia, immunised children may get whooping cough because the vaccine is not 100 per cent protective and because they are exposed to lots of other children and adults coughing whooping cough germs on them. In the United Kingdom nowadays, immunised children do not get whooping cough because almost everyone has been immunised and the resultant herd immunity protects the whole population.

Is it futile to immunise your baby against whooping cough in Australia, then? No. First, immunised children unlucky enough to catch whooping cough get milder disease than unimmunised children. And the '100 day cough', as the Chinese call whooping cough, is a vivid word picture for a disease that causes the child to cough and vomit day and night for over three months, with predictable dire consequences to the health of the child and the wellbeing of the whole exhausted family. Second, levels of whooping cough immunisation are rising in Australia and, when herd immunity levels are achieved, whooping cough will die down again in Australia.

Measles

Measles is a disease that is often misunderstood by the public. It is often perceived by parents and even by some health care professionals as a mild disease, whereas in fact it:

- has killed more Australian children (140) in the last 25 years than all other vaccine-preventable diseases combined, and;

- leaves up to 30 children a year permanently brain-damaged. Even in healthy children, measles often causes a severe illness with pneumonia developing in 2 in every 100 children and convulsions in 1 in every 200.

Some children who have been immunised still get measles. Does this mean that measles vaccine does not work? The answer is similar to that for whooping cough. A single dose of measles vaccine protects 95 to 98 per cent of children, and they will never catch wild-type measles. But no vaccine is 100 per cent effective, and measles is one of the most contagious of all childhood illnesses. In a school or day care centre, most children will have been immunised against measles, a few not. If one unimmunised child catches measles, the other unimmunised children will almost certainly catch measles. But so will 2–5 per cent of immunised children: the vaccine is 95–98 per cent protective, but this means 2–5 per cent of immunised children do not make enough anti-measles antibody to prevent a later infection and are therefore susceptible to catching measles. But their immune system is sufficiently primed by the vaccination to cope much more effectively with the later infection.

There is a paradox here. In an outbreak of measles in a school, it may be that about half the cases of measles occur in children who had been immunised. The anti-immunisation lobby has used this to argue that measles immunisation is useless, only 50 per cent effective. But this is wrong. Say there are 1000 children in a school, 950 have been immunised against measles, 50 not. Of the 950 immunised children, say, 95 per cent are protected, but 5 per cent are non-responders and still susceptible. 5 per cent of 950 is about 47. A measles outbreak occurs in the school. The 50 children who were never immunised will catch measles, but so will the 47 immunised non-responders. So 47, or just under half, of the total 97 who caught measles had been immunised. Is the vaccine 50 per cent effective? No, it is still 95 per cent effective, but because most children had been immunised there was a relatively large pool of immunised non-responders. (Non-responder means not making enough antibody to prevent a later infection. But vaccination has 'primed' their immune system so that they cope much better with the later infection.)

134

The paradox then is that the higher the proportion of children in the school who have been immunised, the greater the number of immunised non-responders, and so the greater the proportion of measles cases in an outbreak who have been immunised. If only half the school had been immunised there would be 500 immunised and 500 not. Of the 500 immunised against measles, 5 per cent or 25 would be susceptible non-responders. In an outbreak the 500 unimmunised children would catch measles, but only 25 non-responders.

Most industrialised countries have adopted a second dose of measles vaccine, often as measles-mumps-rubella (MMR) vaccine at school entry or during high school. This is done to try to prevent school outbreaks of measles that continue to occur. But these occur because of a few unimmunised children, not because measles vaccine does not work.

Polio

Most parents in Australia perceive polio (paralytic poliomyelitis) as a serious disease, but one from the past. They have heard stories of outbreaks of polio in Australia in the 1950s, but they have never seen anyone with polio except in photographs or on television.

Polio is certainly disappearing from the world, as a result of a widespread campaign of polio immunisation promoted by the World Health Organization. This programme aimed to eradicate poliomyelitis from the world by the year 2000. Remarkable progress towards achieving this goal has been made (see Chapter 7), but it will take a little longer than the year 2000.

There are some religious or cultural groups that are opposed to all immunisations. Their children are otherwise healthy, well-nourished and get plenty of exercise. There have been outbreaks of paralytic polio in these religious groups, as well as outbreaks of other vaccine-preventable diseases such as measles and whooping cough. Polio outbreaks have occurred in the last decade in the Amish in the USA, and in fundamental Protestant sects in the Netherlands. These outbreaks affected only the religious groups, and did not spread to their well-immunised neighbours or schoolmates. The outbreaks of poliomyelitis in these groups provide compelling evidence for the efficacy of vaccines and for the dangers of not immunising.

Diphtheria

Diphtheria is a dreaded disease which kills children by choking them to death because of a thick grey membrane which forms in their throat, or by damaging their heart irrevocably. It is highly contagious and has killed thousands of children and young adults a year in countries throughout the world. Since diphtheria immunisation became available, diphtheria has almost totally disappeared from industrialised countries (see Table 5.1). In many developed countries, most infectious disease specialists have never seen a case. The break-up of the USSR into the Confederation of Independent States (CIS) in the early 1990s, together with social upheavals which have adversely affected preparation and delivery of vaccines, led to a drastic fall in immunisation levels. The resulting diphtheria epidemic has been disastrous, with over 150,000 cases in the 1990s in the CIS and over 1,500 deaths. The recent outbreak of diphtheria in Russia is a clear warning that if levels of immunisation were to fall in other countries, diphtheria would return and would cause death and disability as in the past.

Haemophilus influenzae type b

The use of the new 'conjugate' vaccines against *Haemophilus influenzae* type b (Hib) has been a great success story. Hib is a bacterium which can cause bacterial meningitis in children, as well as other potentially life-threatening diseases such as septicaemia, pneumonia, epiglottitis and osteomyelitis. Prior to immunisation it was the commonest cause of bacterial meningitis in Europe, North America and Australasia. In Australia 20 children died from Hib disease each year and 30 who recovered from meningitis were left brain-damaged. Vaccines became available in the late 1980s and their introduction has seen a massive reduction and sometimes even the disappearance of Hib disease within three years in all countries in which it is in routine use. The more than 90 per cent reduction in Hib disease in Australia is shown in Figure 5.3. The vaccine is very safe, with an extremely low rate of side effects, and highly efficacious. It is not a live organism, but consists of the outer sugar coat of the Hib bacterium joined (conjugated) to a protein 'carrier', such as diphtheria or tetanus toxoid.

Parents naturally want to make their own choice about vaccination. Most parents would like a lot of information about vaccines. Either they have not seen the information available from the Health Department, or they want additional information. Many parents would like time to discuss their concerns about immunisation with a knowledgeable health care professional who will talk frankly and honestly about the risks and benefits of vaccines, and not simply dismiss their fears out of hand.

We hope this book, which provides a broader analysis of vaccines and vaccination, will go some way to providing this additional information. Readers are also encouraged to read Chapter 11 and the Epilogue which give extra information about the potential of immunisation procedures to control or clear some non-communicable diseases, as well as infections. In addition, the Epilogue raises the question of whether vaccination is in fact a right and not just a choice.

Table 8.2   Questions and answers about immunisation

Q1. *Are vaccinations safe?*
A.   Not 100 per cent safe, but most of the adverse reactions due to vaccines are relatively minor and reversible. Serious adverse reactions to vaccines are extremely rare. In contrast, serious complications of the diseases are many hundreds of times more common.

Q2. *Isn't it true that most diseases being prevented by vaccines, like measles, are mild and a normal part of growing up?*
A.   Most children will recover without long-term complications from diseases like measles and whooping cough. A significant minority, however, will get serious, potentially life-threatening complications such as pneumonia and encephalitis. Even in developed countries, these will result in deaths and brain damage.

Q3. *Isn't it correct that infectious diseases were disappearing before vaccines were available?*
A.   The disappearance of some diseases, like tuberculosis, from developed countries owes much more to improvements in living conditions than immunisation. Highly infectious agents, like whooping cough, recur as soon as immunisation levels fall, and are only kept at bay by immunisation.

Q4. *Can't I protect my children against infectious diseases by keeping them healthy?*
A.   Good nutrition and a healthy lifestyle are important in protecting against infection. Malnourished children are at greatly increased risk of complications from infection. Unfortunately, however, infectious agents will not only infect malnourished children, but can cause devastating complications to previously healthy, well-nourished children.

Q5. *Don't diseases occur despite immunisation?*
A.   Vaccines are rarely 100 per cent effective, so cases of measles and whooping cough occur despite widespread vaccination, and some cases occur in immunised children. However, *most* immunised children are completely protected—they do not get infected at all. Those immunised children who nevertheless get infected are relatively protected, that is, their disease is milder than if they were unimmunised. And some diseases have been completely eradicated by immunisation (e.g. smallpox) or will soon be eradicated (e.g. polio).

Q6. *Do vaccines cause asthma, allergy, autism, AIDS, cancer or bowel disease?*
A.   No. All these conditions are equally common in unimmunised children. Indeed, hepatitis B vaccine, by protecting against chronic hepatitis B infection, actually reduces the risk of liver cancer.

Q7. *Do vaccines overload the immune system?*
A.   No, the immune system is designed, from birth, to cope with thousands of new substances (antigens) each day. Vaccines represent a tiny proportion of the foreign substances that the immune system recognises and to which the body responds. Live measles vaccine is the only vaccine that may briefly suppress the immune system, and much less so and for a shorter time than natural measles infection. Some natural infections such as HIV/AIDS and malaria can do great damage to the immune system.

Q8. *Can vaccines be contaminated with other viruses?*
A.   Early polio vaccines were contaminated with a monkey virus. There is no evidence that this caused serious harm in recipients. Modern vaccines are free from such contamination.

Q9. *Do vaccines contain human fetal tissue?*
A.   Rubella and varicella viruses are grown on 'immortalised' cell lines, cells which can be grown again and again. These cell lines originally came from human fetal lung tissue many years ago. The Catholic church has no ethical problem with the use of such cells to grow vaccine viruses.

Q10. *Are the additives in vaccines toxic?*
A.   Some vaccines contain aluminium (alum) as an 'adjuvant' to boost the immune response to the target antigen. Alum causes local reactions in a small minority of vaccine recipients. There is a minuscule amount of preservative in some vaccines, which clinical trials have shown to be safe.

II

The way ahead

The previous chapters have dealt with current vaccines, the way they work, their efficacy and their safety. The next three chapters look to some of the latest developments in this area but especially to the future uses of this technology. In recent years there have been striking advances in the study and development of vaccines, which is fortunate as the world continues to be faced with emerging and re-emerging diseases. In a period of less than two decades, HIV/AIDS has become the greatest viral killer of human beings. As we learn more about the mammalian, and especially the human immune system, our ability to make practical use of that knowledge also increases. Chapter 10 outlines new approaches to the development of vaccines against three diseases of global importance and Chapter 12 looks at the encouraging progress now being made in the therapy of non-communicable diseases, cancer and some auto-immune diseases.

9

New approaches to vaccine development and immunisation practices

Twenty to 30 years ago, the number of pharmaceutical companies producing vaccines was diminishing. Since that time, there has been a turnaround with the appearance of increasing numbers of (often) small new biotechnology companies with interest in this area. There may be several reasons for this. As detailed in Chapter 7, the success of the Smallpox Eradication Campaign and the major efforts being made to eradicate poliomyelitis and measles have boosted the image of vaccination. Secondly, the emergence of diseases like AIDS, the growing antibiotic resistance of other infectious agents such as tuberculosis, and the continuing failure to make an impact upon long-term global problems such as malaria have provided a further stimulus to research. Thirdly, advances in biotechnology and the ability to manipulate the immune system have provided new opportunities to design novel types of vaccines.

The current vaccines are predominantly of three types (Chapter 3):

1 *Live attenuated infectious agents.* This approach of using live but weakened forms of the native infectious agent has been particularly successful for viral infections. It also holds promise for bacterial vaccines but the procedures used so far for production have been time-consuming and tedious.
2 *Inactivated, whole organisms,* for both viruses and bacteria. This approach has generally been reasonably successful.
3 *Subunit preparations,* consisting of one or a few proteins or glycoproteins of the agent, or carbohydrate (sugar) sequences conjugated (joined) to a protein 'carrier' which provides the necessary T cell help. This approach has been effective with a number of bacterial vaccines, such as the diphtheria and tetanus toxoids and the *H. influenzae* type b (Hib) vaccine and more recently, the acellular pertussis vaccine. For nearly 20 years, the hepatitis B virus vaccine remained the only licensed subunit vaccine made using recombinant DNA technology (in this case, introducing DNA coding for an antigen into a cell, so that the cell will now produce that antigen), but a genetically engineered subunit vaccine to control tick-borne Lyme disease was licensed in the USA in 1998.

NEW APPROACHES TO VACCINE DEVELOPMENT

Numerous new approaches to vaccine development are being pursued and tested for the ability of the product to induce a strong immune response. Five in particular have attracted a lot of attention and these will be described. It is quite possible that one or two of the others will also lead to the development of useful vaccines.

The first approach is to develop vaccines which are composed only of those sequences which, when recognised by B and T lymphocytes, lead to the induction of protective immune responses. Generally, these are peptide sequences consisting of 'strings' of amino acids (the building blocks of proteins), so such a preparation is often called a 'peptide-based' vaccine. The second is to 'aggregate' protein subunit preparations in different ways so that they induce an enhanced response. The third is to make live attenuated viral or bacterial vaccines by a more reproducible technique, such as weakening the organism by the deletion of specific nucleic acid sequences. The fourth is to modify the best of our existing live attenuated vaccines so that they also express nucleic acid sequences coding for important antigens from one or more other infectious agents. In this way, the attenuated preparation is used as a *vector* for the other foreign antigens. These are sometimes called chimeric vaccines because they 'imitate' a chimera, the beast of Greek mythology which was made up of parts taken from various animals. The fifth approach, which is quite revolutionary, is to immunise with nucleic acid coding for the important antigens. These will be discussed in turn.

PEPTIDE-BASED (AND THEIR EQUIVALENT) VACCINES

Researchers discovered that a vaccine might contain only those parts of the proteins or carbohydrate which were recognised directly by the receptors on B and T lymphocytes. Thus, it would contain only those sequences from proteins or carbohy-drates (B cell epitopes) at the surface of the infectious agent which were recognised by antibodies which could neutralise the infectivity of the agent, whether it be a virus, bacterium or parasite. Second, it would also contain a number of those amino acid sequences (T cell epitopes) in any of the proteins which were recognised by CD4+ or CD8+ T lymphocytes. Sometimes, a particular sequence might be long enough to contain several, possibly overlapping, T cell epitopes.

Potential advantages of this approach

The reason for taking this approach was the belief that such preparations should be very safe to use. First, the preparation would be synthesised in the laboratory or factory rather than prepared from an infectious agent. Second, it would correspond to less than 10 per cent of the sequences in the intact infectious agent. Infection by some viruses or bacteria can cause autoim-mune reactions (reactions against self proteins) because some of their peptide sequences are similar to those in some host proteins. This approach would minimise that risk. However, such preparations have generally resulted in a very weak immune response, that is, they are poorly immunogenic. This is overcome by administering the preparation with an adjuvant, a preparation which enhances its ability to induce a strong immune response. The only adjuvant currently licensed for worldwide human use is alum, containing aluminium and potassium salts. It has been given to a billion or more children when immunising against diphtheria and tetanus and is quite safe. It induces a good type 2 T cell response leading to high antibody levels (Chapter 4). But for some vaccines, a type 1 T cell response is more desirable. Many different types of adjuvants will do this; most so far have been shown to be safe, but none has yet been licensed for general use. Some will be in the not-too-distant future.

Potential disadvantages of this approach

Apart from the fact that several administrations of such vaccines may be needed to induce a protective immune response, they are also likely to be relatively expensive. This approach has one other significant limitation. The idea of linking together T cell epitopes as part of a vaccine (called the 'string-of-beads' or 'poly-epitope' approach) is quite valid (as will be seen in Chapter 10), because the peptides bind directly to major histocompatibility complex proteins. But as stressed in Chapter 4, the antigen-binding sites of infectivity-neutralising antibodies recognise a 'three dimensional shape', usually of an intact protein or polysaccharide as it occurs on the surface of the virus, bacterium or parasite. The shape of the isolated peptide, once it is free of the 'constraints' imposed by the rest of the protein, may be quite different to its shape as part of the protein. This is illustrated in Figure 9.1. As a result, the antibody made to the peptide-based vaccine may bind poorly to the intact virus or bacterium and fail to neutralise its infectivity. One example is the attempt to make a vaccine to the immunodeficiency virus, HIV, as will be discussed in the following Chapter. This has been less of a problem when the B lymphocyte epitope is a carbohydrate structure, on, for example, the surface of some (encapsulated) bacteria.

Though there will be some situations where this approach may be quite successful, it is unlikely to become widely used.

THE USE OF SUBUNIT PREPARATIONS

These will continue to be used in some cases. The protein antigen itself can be presented in different ways, all involving

144

Figure 9.1   Examples of continuous (linear) amino acid sequences (peptides) seen by the antigen-binding site of an antibody.

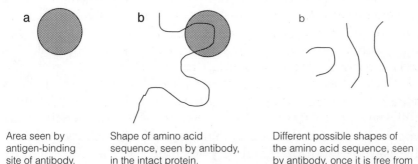

Area seen by antigen-binding site of antibody.

Shape of amino acid sequence, seen by antibody, in the intact protein.

Different possible shapes of the amino acid sequence, seen by antibody, once it is free from the influence of the rest of the protein molecule.

a degree of aggregation of the protein. Sometimes, it can be aggregated to form particles, some of which may be virus-like (VLPs). It can be incorporated into a particle-sized structure called an immunostimulating complex (ISCOM). Or it can be enclosed in a lipid membrane, called a liposome, which readily fuses with a cell membrane. Each of these approaches has been used with some success in different model systems.

THE DEVELOPMENT OF LIVE, ATTENUATED VIRAL AND BACTERIAL VACCINES BY SPECIFIC GENE DELETION TECHNOLOGY

Most of the vaccines of this nature in Tables 3.1 and 3.2, were made by passaging the infectious agent many times in different cell cultures and/or in selected hosts. Clearly, the technique worked but it was tedious, time-consuming and the outcome could not be guaranteed in advance. Once it became possible to sequence the genome, RNA or DNA, of the infectious agent, virus or bacteria, the selective removal of certain nucleic acid sequences, such as those coding for particular proteins with known undesirable activities became possible. An attenuated strain of vaccinia virus, called NYVAC (New York vaccinia) was made by selectively deleting DNA coding for particular proteins of the vaccinia virus, amounting to about 10 per cent of the total DNA. The attenuated strain was very much less pathogenic (causing disease) for mice compared to the parental strain, but retained the ability to induce a good immune response. The 'space' previously occupied by the deleted DNA sequences could then be 'filled' by segments of DNA coding for antigens of other agents, as described below.

A similar approach is being used to make attenuated bacteria for use as vaccines, such as salmonella.

Many bacteria, including Salmonella, contain a single gene which codes for a protein, called DNA adenine methylase (abbreviated to Dam). When this gene in salmonella was knocked out, the bacteria completely lost the ability to cause disease but retained the ability to induce a powerful immune response in mice. It seems possible that in many bacteria a single gene might control the activities of many other genes involved in inducing disease. If this result can be duplicated, an extraordinarily simple way of making powerful but safe bacterial vaccines for human use is within reach.

USING EXISTING VACCINES AS 'VECTORS' OF ANTIGENS FROM OTHER DISEASE AGENTS

The rationale behind this approach is twofold. First, there are some highly effective live attenuated vaccines, especially against viral infections. Can they become even more useful than they are now? Second, we have some infections due to viruses or bacteria for which, for one reason or another, there has been great difficulty in making an effective vaccine. If the identity of important antigen(s), say the targets for infectivity-neutralising antibody is known, can the DNA (or RNA, depending on the vector) coding for these antigens be inserted into the genome of the live vaccine virus or bacteria? The technique is shown in Figure 9.2. When susceptible cells in the host are infected by the chimeric viruses or bacteria, proteins coded for by the inserted nucleic acid would be produced. These would initiate an immune response which should protect hosts later exposed to the agent which was the source of the inserted nucleic acid.

This approach was first described in the early 1980s by two Americans, Bernie Moss and Enzo Paoletti and, very quickly, a group headed by David Boyle was established to further research it in the John Curtin School in Canberra. The group was

Figure 9.2   The technique of making a chimeric (recombinant) virus.

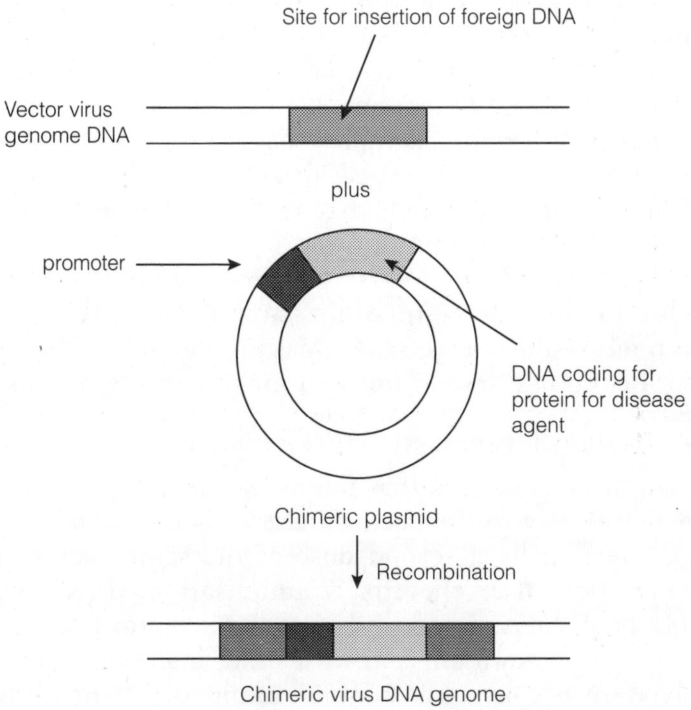

Site for insertion of foreign DNA

Vector virus
genome DNA

plus

promoter

DNA coding for
protein for disease
agent

Chimeric plasmid

Recombination

Chimeric virus DNA genome

supported by the CSIRO (Commonwealth Scientific & Industrial Research Organisation) as an adjunct to their Animal Health Division at Geelong, which had a major interest in vaccines to control infections in commercially important farm animals.

Potential advantages of this approach

First, the efficacy and safety of some of our current live attenuated vaccines, demonstrated over many years, would be exploited even more. Second, only one or two administrations of the modified vaccine should be required to yield a good immune response. Third, this preparation should induce both good antibody and T lymphocyte responses, including cytotoxic T lymphocytes. Depending upon the size of the vector being used, it is possible to insert DNA coding for antigens from several different viruses. This has been done with poxviruses.

Fourth (and somewhat later), Ian Ramshaw in the John Curtin School, and Bernie Moss (USA) developed the idea of also incorporating in the chimeric vector, nucleic acid coding for important cytokines (immune-modulating molecules, see Chapter 4), such as the different interleukins or gamma interferon. This would enable, for example, specific enhancement of the immune response in a desired direction, of either antibody production or type 1 T lymphocyte responses when the modified construct was used to immunise a host.

The attenuated live virus vaccines used in the WHO Expanded Programme of Immunization are relatively inexpensive to produce on a large scale. Making modified preparations as described above should not add greatly to the expense.

Potential disadvantages of this approach

The main disadvantage is that following the first use of a vector like this, antibody to the vector antigens is made and this may prevent infection by a second dose of the same vector, if it is given too soon after the first immunisation. This could be particularly disadvantageous if the same vector was used at different times to immunise against other infections. Those (fortunately) rare people with a faulty immune system, (immunocompromised), can become seriously ill if exposed to the natural disease agent. But the use of attenuated or chimeric, attenuated infectious agents have caused little trouble in this respect. Sometimes, the immune response to the foreign antigens coded for by the inserted nucleic acid is not as strong as hoped for, but this technology is becoming very popular as will be seen in the following Chapter.

Table 9.1 lists some of the different viruses and bacteria being used as vectors of the DNA of other infectious disease in experimental studies. Some constructs are undergoing testing for efficacy and safety in clinical trials. None so far is licensed for use as a vaccine for humans, but that time is not far off.

GENETIC IMMUNISATION, OR THE USE OF 'NAKED' DNA FOR VACCINATION

In 1990, J. A. Wolff (USA) was carrying out experiments in mice on gene transfer by injecting the DNA coding for the gene into

Table 9.1   Some live, attenuated viruses and bacteria under investigation as vectors of nucleic acid coding for protective antigens from other infectious agents

Viruses

Poxviruses—Vaccinia; Ankara strain; NYVAC (New York vaccinia); fowlpox; canarypox
Other viruses—Adeno; varicella; polio; influenza

Bacteria.

M. bovis (BCG); Salmonella strains

Notes: The main viruses used are members of the pox group. They are very large viruses, and about 10 per cent of DNA can be excised from their genome without affecting their ability to act as a vector. This means that DNA coding for perhaps ten different antigens, say three or four from three different disease agents, can be inserted into the genome of the modified virus.

Vaccinia is the basis of the smallpox vaccine, but in the past it has given a significant level of side reactions. For this reason, it may not be used widely in humans again. Ankara is a strain of vaccinia that was developed during the smallpox eradication campaign and, like NYVAC, is much less reactogenic than vaccinia. Fowlpox and canarypox viruses are members of the avipox group. These viruses infect mammalian cells, the antigens encoded in the DNA are expressed but infectious virus is not made. In effect therefore, these strains are potentially very safe vectors. The other viruses quoted, especially adenovirus, will serve particular purposes. For example, there are multiple strains of the adenovirus so that if repeated administrations were required, different strains could be used on each occasion to avoid neutralisation of each dose of vector by pre-existing antibody.

BCG, the attenuated form of *M. bovis* and the basis of the tuberculosis vaccine, is theoretically attractive to use as a vector, but to date, the results obtained have been variable. In contrast, the use of salmonella strains has fairly consistently given encouraging results (see main text).

mouse muscle. As well as answering the questions he was asking in his experiment, he observed that it would be of interest to see if the mouse made an immune response to the proteins coded for by the foreign DNA. Two years later, this was shown to be the case; mice made a persisting antibody response of the anticipated specificity. It was soon found that a comprehensive T cell response also occurred, including the formation of cytotoxic T lymphocytes.

Bacterial plasmids are double-stranded circles of DNA (Chapter 1). They replicate independently of the chromosomal DNA in bacteria and can be transferred between bacteria. Figure 9.3 illustrates the technique of making a chimeric plasmid. The DNA coding for antigens from an infectious agent is inserted into the plasmid behind a 'promoter' which ensures strong expression of the inserted DNA once the plasmid enters a host cell. The plasmid preparation can be injected into muscle where it enters the myofibrils (muscle cells) and these cells then

Figure 9.3 The technique of making a chimeric plasmid.

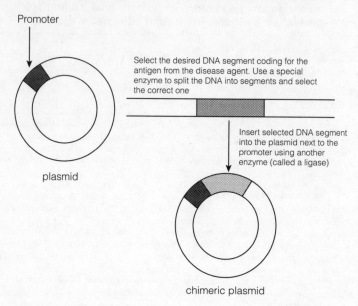

The chimeric plasmid is introduced into the bacterial host. The bacteria are grown up to the required amount and the plasmids are then harvested.

probably act as a DNA depot. It seems very likely that some plasmids are taken up by other cells such as dendritic cells which are particularly good at presenting antigens to the immune system. This would be one reason for the observed good immune response.

Another approach has been to coat very tiny gold beads with the plasmids and, using a 'gene-gun', to 'shoot' them into the skin. Some plasmids are then picked up by local dendritic cells and taken off to the draining lymph nodes where the immune response is initiated. This is a more economical method than by direct injection but, as will be discussed in the second half of this chapter, there are also other possibilities.

Potential advantages of this approach

The first important feature of this approach is that immunisation with DNA induces a broad immune response similar to that given by the original infectious agent, or by an attenuated strain. However, as the DNA is non-infectious, it should not cause disease. One additional benefit is that there should be no risk of inducing disease in people who are immunocompromised.

The second point is that, like the peptide-based or subunit approach to making vaccines, the immune response is confined to the protein(s) coded for by the inserted DNA in the plasmid. Third, the pre-existing presence of antigen-specific antibody should not interfere with the induction of immunity to the nominated protein. Thus, for example, it will be recalled (Chapters 3, 7) that the current measles vaccine cannot be given to an infant younger than nine months of age because of the presence of maternally derived anti-measles antibody; a new measles vaccine made using this new technology could be administered to infants in endemic countries shortly after birth. Fourth, there is so far no indication that the host makes antibody to the injected DNA itself, so that the same host could be sequentially immunised with plasmids containing DNA coding for different foreign antigens, a very important advantage.

Finally, plasmids, once constructed to include the appropriate DNA coding for foreign proteins, are propagated in bacteria. Producing bacteria in large quantities is simple and inexpensive, so again, DNA vaccines should be quite affordable for the consumer. The plasmids are also heat stable and robust, highly desirable properties for a vaccine.

In the relatively short time since this approach to vaccine development 'hit the headlines', many experiments have been carried out mainly in mice but more recently in monkeys and chimpanzees with plasmids containing DNA coding for antigens from a wide variety of infectious agents. The experiments have shown that immunisation with DNA can give protection against many infectious agents. Some clinical trials are already in progress. They all point to the conclusion that in the early years of the new millennium, DNA vaccines are likely to become a reality.

Potential disadvantages of this approach

Other than concerns about safety and the fact that in most cases, several administrations of the vaccine are required, there are no obvious disadvantages to this approach. When a new technology like this first appears, authorities associated with monitoring adverse reactions to vaccines make a list of possibilities that can be looked for when the product is tested at the experimental and clinical trial stages. For example, if some of the DNA in the plasmid became incorporated into the host's chromosomes, it is theoretically conceivable that it might interfere with the usual pattern of expression of host DNA. Or frequent administration of plasmids might cause the formation of anti-DNA antibodies; these could prevent the DNA from being effective. So far, there is no indication that anything of this nature happens.

NEWER APPROACHES TO VACCINATION PRACTICES

There are several developments which are of particular interest. These are detailed below.

Enhancing immune responses at mucosal surfaces

A glance at Tables 3.1 and 3.2 shows one inescapable fact. Most natural infections by agents for which vaccines are available infect via a mucosal site, especially the respiratory route, whereas most corresponding vaccines are administered by injection. One of the reasons for this was that administering an antigen by a mucosal route often gave only a short-lived immune response. Three or more doses of the oral polio vaccine (OPV, the live attenuated strains) are required in order to induce a lasting immune response.

The systemic immune system, involving the spleen and some lymph nodes, has some different characteristics compared to the mucosal system. The latter has its own special form of antibody, secretory immunoglobulin A (s.IgA), whereas IgG, IgM and IgE characterise the systemic system. In the mid-1970s, it was found by John Bienenstock and colleagues (Canada) that there was a 'common mucosal system'—that immunising at one mucosal surface could result in the appearance of a protective immune response at another mucosal site. For example, the adenovirus causes an acute respiratory infection. An adenovirus vaccine was made some years ago for use by the USA armed forces. It is given orally but protects against a respiratory infection! We now know that this interchange between different mucosal sites is not quite as general as was first thought. It mainly involves the traffic of T lymphocytes, activated by immunisation at one mucosal site, to other mucosal sites. The interest in this field is such that the study of mucosal immunology has over the years become a major international discipline.

The major mucosal sites and the 'supply' of lymphoid tissues draining those sites are listed in Table 9.2. The gut and especially the rectum (the region of the gastrointestinal tract closest to the anus) are very well endowed with associated lymphoid tissues. There is a special mechanism in the gut to deal with soluble foreign antigens, especially from the breakdown of foods. The quantity and variety of these are so great that potentially, if an immune response was made against food proteins, we would be in serious trouble and might starve to death. Instead a mechanism has developed in the gut whereby a state of tolerance is induced against soluble proteins in general (the body cannot distinguish between proteins from food or any other source). To induce a good immune response, the foreign antigens should be administered as particles (like viruses or bacteria) or mimicking such agents, or given with a powerful adjuvant (a substance or formulation which stimulates the immune system). Similarly, the respiratory tract is well supplied with associated lymphoid tissues, as there are many airborne infectious agents.

Prevention and control of sexually transmitted diseases

A number of bacteria colonise the vagina, and these together with a slightly acid environment, help to keep that area healthy. Although during an infection, some lymphoid tissue can develop in the upper part of the female reproductive tract (above the cervix), the vagina itself is poorly supplied with asssociated lymphoid tissue. Why is this so? The answer is simple. Every

Table 9.2   The major mucosal sites, route of contact and the associated lymphoid tissues

Mucosal site	Route for contact	Associated lymphoid tissues
The gut (gastro-intestinal tract)	Oral	Peyer's patches, appendix
Rectal	Anus	Very well supplied
Bronchus (lung, tonsillar tissues)	Nose	Well supplied
Genito-urinary tract	Vagina	Poorly supplied

time there is active heterosexual intercourse, about half a billion sperm are deposited in the vagina. For the female immune system, this could be a substantial dose of foreign (male) antigen, especially as most sperm rapidly die in the vagina due to the hostile (for sperm) environment. Of the huge number of sperm deposited in the vagina, about 30 reach the female ovum. Taken together with the fact that there is also a limited number of times a year when fertilisation can occur, the success versus failure rate of our reproductive system is very finely balanced. If an anti-sperm antibody response was generally induced by the frequent deposition of sperm, the whole reproductive system of mammals, especially humans, would fail. In fact, some women do make anti-sperm antibodies and they become infertile. One additional complication is that the immune response in the female reproductive tract is influenced by the estrous (hormonal) cycle. These different factors may contribute to the success rate of infection by some sexually transmitted diseases (STDs), such as gonorrhoea, syphilis, genital herpes and chlamydia to name a few. As reported in Chapter 5, there was in 1995 an alarming increase in the number of new cases of STDs worldwide, but especially in some developing countries.

What might be the best route of immunisation to prevent or control infection by STDs? Recent work has shown some success if the vaccine is injected to a site adjacent to the iliac lymph nodes which are close to and 'drain' (are linked to) the female reproductive tract. Attempts to provoke a protective immune response in the reproductive tract by oral administration of a vaccine have given variable results. But increasing numbers of reports are showing that immunisation via the respiratory tract can lead to a good immune response in the female reproductive tract. For example, a chimeric adenovirus containing DNA coding for a herpes virus antigen administered intranasally to female mice induced a strong antibody response, both s.IgA and IgG, to herpes virus in the reproductive tract.

Will immunisation via a mucosal surface become more popular in vaccination programmes?

Most people who work in this area would probably answer yes to this question. In the case of subunit or peptide-based preparations, it would be essential to administer the preparation with an adjuvant which was effective at a mucosal surface. Currently, the one most used in experimental studies is the toxin protein from the cholera bacterium (cholera toxin, or CT). It is very effective at inducing a strong antibody response to the vaccine protein, (i.e., a type 2 T lymphocyte response—see Chapter 4). It is debatable whether CT will be recommended for general human use. At present, if a type 1 T lymphocyte response is desired, it is not clear what adjuvant will be most effective, other than to say that one might not be necessary if plasmids were used for vaccination.

The use of live vectors provides extra opportunities. Most work has been done with the different poxviruses, including the two avipoxes, fowlpox and canarypox (Table 9.1) which infect but do not replicate in mammalian cells.

There are now numerous reports on the use of live, attenuated salmonella bacterial strains as vectors of DNA coding for other antigens. The vector containing the plasmids is given orally and is adsorbed to and taken up by M cells, a special type of cell present at the surface of the gut mucosa. The bacteria travel to the draining lymphoid tissue, called the Peyer's patches, where the particular form of attenuation employed in modifying the bacteria results in their death. One particular example is of special interest. The bacterium *Listeria monocytogenes* causes sporadic outbreaks of disease, especially in the newborn and elderly, which can be fatal. DNA plasmids containing genes coding for some Listerial antigens were grown in *Escherichia coli* bacteria, isolated and transferred to the *Salmonella typhi* Aro A mutant bacteria (which is close to registration as a medical vaccine). When the chimeric bacteria were fed *once* orally to mice, there was a surprisingly strong immune response, so powerful that the mice were protected from death when challenged with a potentially lethal dose of listeria bacteria. Further findings suggested that when these chimeric bacteria died in the lymphoid tissue, they were phagocytosed (absorbed) by macrophages and dendritic cells, which are good antigen-presenting cells (APCs). In other words, this experimental approach seemed to result in the *direct delivery* of the plasmids to APCs, and this could explain why a good protective effect after immunisation was achieved.

Clinical trials are underway to establish whether encouraging results like this in mice can be reproduced in humans.

Sequential vaccination

It is the traditional practice that when multiple doses of a vaccine are required, the same vaccine is used for each dose administered. In the early 1990s in many studies in the USA on the development of an HIV (AIDS) vaccine, it was commonly found that the envelope protein in particular was poorly immunogenic—repeated immunisations still gave only a mediocre antibody response. Two of the preparations available at that time were a chimeric vaccinia virus containing DNA coding for the HIV envelope protein, gp160, and a subunit preparation of gp160. By administering the vaccinia construct first to human volunteers followed by the subunit preparation, it was found that an enhanced antibody response occurred, greater than that seen when two successive doses of each preparation were given to volunteers.

Ian Ramshaw and his colleagues at the John Curtin School of Medical Research had been working with a chimeric fowlpox virus containing the DNA coding for an influenza viral protein. Ian rapidly acquired the DNA technology when it first became available and made a plasmid containing the DNA coding for the same influenza viral protein. The team then asked the question—if mice were injected first with the plasmid and later with the chimeric fowlpox preparation, would there be an enhanced antibody response compared to that of mice injected only with the chimeric fowlpox? The answer was clearcut—mice receiving DNA followed by the virus gave antibody titres (concentrations) up to 50 times higher than those receiving only the chimeric virus. The result suggested that the DNA preparation was particularly good at priming mice for an immune response!

In 1998, there were four reports showing a similar enhancing effect. In each case, animals were injected first with a DNA preparation followed by a chimeric poxvirus construct. The aims were to generate a strong cytotoxic T lymphocyte (CTL) response. Andrew McMichael and colleagues from the Institute of Molecular Medicine, Oxford, using HIV antigens and Adrian Hill and colleagues (also from the Institute) using malaria antigens also found that very strong CTL responses were generated

156

in mice in this way. In contrast, if the virus construct was given first followed by the DNA preparation, this enhanced response was not seen! Ian Ramshaw, with Stephen Kent of the Macfarlane Burnet Centre, Melbourne, immunised *M. nemestrima* monkeys first with a DNA construct followed by a fowlpox construct. Each contained antigens from HIV and strong anti-HIV CTL responses were induced. When later challenged with HIV, these monkeys rapidly cleared the infection whereas control (non-immunised) monkeys didn't. It was subsequently reported (Harriet Robinson, USA) that monkeys immunised in a rather similar fashion using first DNA and then fowlpox preparations containing DNA coding for antigens from simian immunodeficiency virus (SIV), protected the animals from death when they were later challenged with a very virulent (lethal) SHIV preparation.

These experiments also confirmed that there is clearly something special about bacterial plasmids. It has been established that bacterial DNA contains some nucleotide sequences which can enhance the immune response to an antigen. When such a mixture was injected systemically or administered intranasally to mice, there was an enhanced immune response. In the latter case, the mucosal IgA response was of the same size as that given when cholera toxin (CT) was used as an adjuvant with the same antigen. But whereas CT induced primarily a Th2 T lymphocyte response (mainly antibody) to the protein, the nucleotide sequence induced as well a Th1 T lymphocyte response, including cytotoxic T lymphocyte activity, to the protein.

FURTHER SURPRISES

Scientific research has the great attraction that simply by trying to satisfy curiosity, quite novel findings can sometimes be made. One fascinating finding is that if an antigen solution including some CT was painted directly on the skin of shaved mice, a reasonable antibody response was obtained. It is too early to predict how applicable this finding may be for medical use, but it suggests the possibility for another less invasive technique for vaccine delivery.

There is one more surprise for those reading this chapter. For generations, plants have been a rich source of medicinal compounds. Now plants may be even more useful, as a means of delivering vaccines. It is possible to introduce into some plant cells the DNA coding for viral antigens such as the hepatitis B surface antigen, HBsAg (a process called DNA transfection of cells). Transgenic tobacco and potato plants made in this way by Charles Arntzen and colleagues (USA) were found to produce lots of the viral antigen. The product could either be isolated and purified from the plant or the plant product (raw potatoes) fed directly to animals. Mice fed this way have made antibodies to the viral antigen. Adding traces of cholera toxin to the potato slices improved the immune response. An alternative approach is to infect plants with a chimeric plant virus—in one case a virus engineered to contain the nucleic acid coding for rabies virus antigens (Hilary Koprowski and colleagues, USA). When the chimeric plant virus or, more simply, leaves from the infected plant, were fed to mice, some of the mice made an immune response which was sufficiently strong to protect them from disease when they were challenged with rabies virus.

Some clinical trials of these plant-derived preparations are underway. In one trial, volunteers ate raw potato slices from transgenic plants which synthesised a toxin from *E. coli*, a bacterium that causes diarrhoea in infants and often in travellers. Both mucosal and systemic anti-toxin immune responses were induced in the volunteers. It has been suggested that bananas would be the ideal 'vector' for such products, especially in developing countries where often the cost of new vaccines may be too high a burden for a local government.

An additional trend is the production in plants of specific antibodies ('plantibodies') for either prophylactic (disease-preventing) or therapeutic uses. In mammals, the production of secretory IgA (sIgA) involves the collaboration between two different cells, B lymphocytes and mucosal epithelial cells. In contrast, the complete molecule has been made in a single tobacco plant cell! In one case (Julian Ma and colleagues, USA), an antibody to the common oral bacterium, *Streptococcus mutans*, which contributes to tooth decay was applied to the teeth in specially cleaned mouths of volunteers. It successfully prevented recolonisation of the mouth by these bacteria for four months. In the future, transgenic plants could be a relatively inexpensive source of such antibodies for topical application.

In this chapter, we have discussed the new approaches to vaccine development. The two which currently hold the greatest promise for wide use in the immediate future are chimeric live vectors, both viruses and bacteria, and the use of DNA plasmids. The latter in particular seems set to revolutionise vaccine development and administration practices in the next 10–15 years. There are more surprises in store, such as the production of some vaccines and antibody preparations in plants.

In the next chapter, we discuss progress in the development of vaccines to several very severe diseases of global importance, beginning with HIV. Will the availability of these new techniques make a difference to this task or are the prospects still not very encouraging?

10

The challenge of making vaccines against HIV, malaria and chlamydia

Most of the effective vaccines available in the world today are against infectious agents which cause acute infections, that is, infections which, if a less-than-lethal dose is given, will be cleared by the host's own immune system. But there are many infectious agents, including many viruses, bacteria and most parasites which cause chronic persisting infections. During evolution, these agents have learnt how to evade the immune system of their host, causing considerable sickness and sometimes a high death rate. In some cases, it may be still possible to make an effective vaccine if there is little or no antigenic variation in the antigen(s) recognised by antibodies which neutralise infectivity. The hepatitis B vaccine is one such example. But if there is considerable variation in the relevant antigen of other infectious agents, then it becomes a more difficult task. In this chapter, we discuss three such agents—HIV (AIDS), *Plasmodium* (malaria) and *Chlamydia trachomatis* (trachoma and pelvic inflammatory disease). These three are listed in Table 1.3 as leading causes of sickness and death in the world. Attempts to make an effective vaccine against these diseases have been ongoing for many years, varying from ten or more for HIV to 30 years or more for malaria. In this chapter, we explain some of the reasons for the lack of success to date and outline current attempts to overcome these difficulties.

HUMAN IMMUNODEFICIENCY VIRUS (HIV)—THE 'CLEVER' VIRUS

AIDS is an emerging disease. It now (1999) seems very likely that it originated from one sub-species of African chimpanzees which have been infected, probably for many generations, with a similar but for them a non-lethal virus, a simian immunodeficiency virus (SIVcpz). It is considered that the virus was transmitted to those men who prepared infected chimps for eating. On at least one occasion since the middle of the twentieth century, the virus adjusted to its new host, man, by rapid and extensive mutation to become in a remarkably short time what we now call HIV type 1. With increased population movement in Africa, modern transport facilities and more sexual freedom, the virus spread within Africa and thence especially to the USA. A very brief history of events since then is as follows:

A sequence of important findings since 1981

1 The disease AIDS, acquired immunodeficiency syndrome, was diagnosed in the USA in 1981–2, initially in homosexual men. The virus could be transmitted by sexual acts, by intravenous drug users, in blood products and from infected mothers to babies.

2 The infectious agent, a retrovirus called human immunodeficiency virus type 1, HIV–1, was isolated in 1983–4. The CD4 molecule on some human T lymphocytes was identified as a receptor for the virus, resulting in infection of that cell. The virus could now be grown in bulk in these cells. However, expression of human CD4 molecules on mouse cells did not allow infection of those cells. This was the first indication that there might be a second receptor for HIV on human cells.

3 The complete nucleotide sequence of the viral RNA was described in 1985. The virus was found to have three major structural proteins, the envelope protein (env), gag and

polymerase (pol) as well as eight regulatory proteins (which control viral replication in cells).

4 Another HIV-like virus, also called SIV, could cause an AIDS-like disease in macaque monkeys, but not in African green monkeys. It is closely related to another human virus, HIV–2, which occurs mainly in west Africa.

5 Advances in knowledge about the structure of the virus and its life cycle were so spectacularly rapid that there was already talk about developing a vaccine as early as 1986–7.

6 By 1987–8, the first warning signs of potential difficulties were appearing. HIV was being isolated from many different cell types, including brain cells, in infected humans. There were the first indications of considerable antigenic variation in the envelope protein. Some anti-viral antibody (which did not neutralise the viral infectivity), could facilitate entry of HIV into macrophages, and thus increase the rate of infection of those cells (a phenomenon called 'immune enhancement of infection'—see the Glossary). High levels of anti-HIV cytotoxic T lymphocytes (CTLs) were found in the blood of many infected people; why didn't they clear the infection?

7 In 1988, it was proposed that because of the increasing indications of great antigenic variation in the envelope protein (on the outside of the virus particle), a vaccine would not be successful unless it could generate a very early strong CTL response before the virus became widely distributed around the body. This might best be achieved by using a chimeric live virus vector, vaccinia, containing the DNA coding for several HIV antigens. At that time and shortly after, lists could be made of some of the features of the virus and of the disease which made HIV a difficult target for vaccine development (Table 10.1).

8 However, the major interested vaccine manufacturers wished to use the envelope protein (env) as the basis of a subunit vaccine, despite the very great variation between different preparations worldwide, and even within a single infected person. They were encouraged by two findings— first, that a powerful anti-envelope antibody (a monoclonal antibody) could protect chimpanzees from a challenge injection of that strain of HIV; and second, that immunising

**Table 10.1   Some features of HIV which obstruct vaccine
development**

The virus
1   Very great antigenic variation
2   The virus infects many different cell types in the body

The infection and disease
1   The infection may be transmitted by infected cells which express viral antigens
     and may produce virus.
3   Viral RNA is copied into a DNA form (copy DNA) which then integrates into
     the host cell genome
4   The virus persists after infection, despite a strong host immune response
5   Crucial cells of the immune system are infected and die, especially CD4+ T
     lymphocytes and dendritic cells. Consequently, a state of immunodeficiency
     occurs
6   Antibodies may enhance infection in cells such as macrophages
7   An affordable and susceptible animal model which, after infection, develops
     disease like the human pattern, is not readily available

---

*   Cells can be latently infected. The viral copy DNA is integrated into the cell's DNA, but is
     not expressed. The body's immune system has no way of knowing that the cell is
     infected. Some time later (weeks, months, years), this cell can be 're-activated' and start
     to produce virus.

chimpanzees with the env protein could protect them from
a later challenge with the same strain of virus. Furthermore,
different env preparations were found to be safe when
administered to volunteers.

9   But when these preparations were submitted for approval to
     undergo a phase III clinical trial (to prevent a natural
     infection) in the mid-1990s, the proposal was not approved.
     Many reasons were given, but two important ones were:

     (i) that antibody from immunised volunteers, though it
         prevented infection by virus grown in T lymphocytes,
         had recently been found not to prevent infection by
         freshly isolated wild-type virus obtained from naturally
         infected people; and
     (ii) that the preparations, as administered, did not induce
         CTL formation.

10   Later studies showed that whereas the envelope protein
     occurred as single molecules on T lymphocyte-grown virus,
     it occurred as groups of three molecules, a trimer, on freshly
     isolated wild-type virus. (This pattern of small groupings of
     identical polymers, often called oligomers, is seen with some

other viruses, such as influenza). Antibody to the envelope trimer was found to neutralise many native strains of HIV. This at last seemed to give strong hope that a vaccine which induced a protective antibody response could be made. In 1998, however, three HIV isolates (from HIV-infected infants) were found which were not neutralised by this antibody. So this approach may be in doubt.

11 In the meantime, it was shown that when attenuated live SIV preparations (with one or more genes deleted) were used to immunise monkeys, they were protected from a later strong challenge with SIV. This seemed very promising, but alas, these preparations have turned out to be unsafe as they caused AIDS in young monkeys. Attenuated strains of HIV have been isolated from some infected people (the first case was in Australia), but it is not clear how long these people may remain disease free. So the approach to make an attenuated live HIV vaccine is now on hold.

12 Then, as predicted, a second receptor for HIV on T lymphocytes was found, a molecule whose normal function is as a receptor for some messenger molecules called chemokines. It was found:

(i) that individuals with defective cellular chemokine receptors *could not be infected with HIV*; and

(ii) that an excess of normal chemokine molecules could also *inhibit infection of cells by HIV*.

It was then established that mouse cells which are engineered to express both human CD4 and the human chemokine receptor could be infected by HIV.

13 This finding has led (1999) to a completely novel approach to HIV vaccine development. A transfected cell expressing the HIV envelope (env) protein (that is, mimicking the virus) was allowed to bind to a cell expressing both the CD4 and the chemokine receptors. When the two cells had fused and both receptors for env were occupied, the complex was chemically 'fixed' so the cells could not separate. Immunising mice with this complex induced antibodies which neutralised the infectivity of nearly every known 'strain' of HIV. It is thought that when the above fusion occurred, the env protein was 'distorted' and kept in that state by the fixation

procedure. This exposed for the first time antigenically conserved sequences against which the new antibodies were made. It is too early to say how practical this approach for developing a strong antibody-inducing HIV vaccine may be.

Will a vaccine inducing mainly or only anti-HIV
cytotoxic T lymphocyte (CTL) formation be effective?

There are 100 or so different potential HIV vaccines under development. Of the seven or eight leading candidates, most induce both antibody and CTL formation. Both responses are desirable. But, as described in Chapter 9, two of these preparations (one Australian, one UK) induce effectively only CTL responses.

Table 10.2 lists the evidence supporting a very important role for CTLs in controlling this infection. Table 10.2A describes four different 'experiments of nature' which support such a concept. These were the identification of five groups of individuals who had been exposed to HIV, who possessed HIV-specific CTLs in their blood, yet no HIV could be isolated or virus-specific serum antibody detected. These include a group of Nairobi prostitutes, a finding which is particularly impressive as the transmission rate of HIV in that area is very high. Presumably, all the individuals in these studies made a strong CTL response after their *first* exposure to the virus (possibly after exposure to only a very low dose of virus). This response cleared the virus and protected these individuals against later infections.

The second part (Table 10.2B) describes some other supporting observations. Generally, HIV-infected individuals who do not progress to AIDS (or progress very slowly) make a strong CTL response which persists. Others who progress more rapidly to AIDS also can make CTL responses but these responses disappear before AIDS occurs. As CTL responses involve the recognition of class I major histocompatibility complex (MHC) antigens (for humans, HLA antigens), one would expect persisting CTL responses to involve (be associated with) some particular HLA specificities and non-persisting responses to involve different HLA specificities. This is precisely what has been found. One possible explanation would be that HLA alleles (specificities) B27 and A32 bind viral peptides which are not

Table 10.2   Evidence that cytotoxic T lymphocytes (CTLs) may control/clear an HIV infection

A   *Detection of HIV-specific CTLs in virus-free, seronegative individuals*
1   In babies born of infected mothers
2   In long-term partners of infected persons
3   In a small proportion of long-term prostitutes in the Gambia and in Nairobi
4   In 7 of 20 health care workers accidentally exposed to infected blood

B   *Other evidence*
5   Long-term, non-progressors to AIDS have strong CTL responses
6   Some HLA class I specificities (HLA B27, A32) are associated with protective effects: others (HLA B35, B39, A24) are associated with rapid progression to disease
7   Temporary killing of CD8 +T lymphocytes in SIV-infected monkeys causes a surge in viral growth (two independent reports in 1998 and 1999)

subject to mutation (are conserved) during the course of the infection; in contrast, the peptides binding to B35, B39 and A24 may be subject to mutation. Finally, if CD8+ T lymphocytes were involved in controlling an HIV infection, their temporary absence in the body would result in a surge of viral growth. This cannot be checked with humans, but using the monkey/SIV model, transfer of anti-CD8+ T lymphocyte antibody to the infected monkeys has this effect. In the temporary absence of CD8+ lymphocytes (CTLs), there was a strong surge in viral growth in the monkeys.

Alternatively, if the vaccination protocol described above does not clear an HIV infection, it should at least reduce the virus load to such an extent that the individual becomes a 'non-progressor' to AIDS, that is, the person, though infected, remains healthy for a longer time and may become less infectious for others.

The above very brief account should give the reader some idea of the trials and tribulations experienced by those involved in HIV vaccine development for the last decade or so. It has been a unique learning experience. There is still a lot of confidence that a vaccine will become available in due course. Particularly for the sake of those living in developing countries where the toll of HIV infection is now enormous and multidrug therapy is not available, we must hope that there will be a successful outcome.

The *Plasmodium* parasite, the agent causing malaria

In contrast to AIDS, malaria is not an emerging disease, but it may now be classified as a re-emerging disease, because of the increasing incidence of drug-resistant parasites during the last few decades. The disease is now so prevalent in large areas of the globe that tourists to some countries must be warned about travelling to those regions.

There are more than 100 *Plasmodium* species that infect different hosts. Four infect humans and of these, *P. falciparum* is the most important. None of the other 96+ infections in different hosts completely mimics the human infection, but some have been helpful as models.

The Plasmodium *life cycle*

There are three stages:

1 Human infection begins when an infected female mosquito injects sporozoites in her saliva through the skin. Within a very short time, sporozoites reach and infect liver cells. They divide and form schizonts, a process which may take up to a week in humans.
2 Each schizont may contain thousands of the next infectious form, merozoites, and upon their release from the liver, the schizonts rupture. Within minutes, the released merozoites infect red blood cells (RBCs). After the release of merozoite progeny from one RBC, fresh RBCs are immediately infected. After several sequential rounds of replication in this way, some of the merozoites differentiate into a sexual form, the gametocyte.
3 When ingested by another biting female mosquito, the gametocytes mate. In time, new sporozoites form, accumulate in the mosquito saliva and the cycle can then begin again.

The infected RBC stage is responsible for the intermittent fevers and malaise which are characteristic of this infection. Immunity to malaria does occur. The death rate of children under five is high, but generally older children and adults survive, though they may have bouts of illness and continually carry the parasite. Sometimes, they are said to be *Plasmodia-tolerant*.

The importance of antibody

Ever since it was shown in 1961 that transfer of antibody from immune persons greatly reduced the level of parasites in infected African children, the accent has been on developing a vaccine which primarily induced protective antibodies. The major aim was to prevent the infection of RBCs (stage 2). Despite great international efforts in this direction over the last 30 years, the results have been relatively disappointing with few products reaching the clinical trial stage. Because of the growing urgency to develop an effective vaccine, an international group, the Multilateral Initiative on Malaria, has been formed with members ranging from scientists to politicians.

Difficulties versus opportunities for developing malaria vaccines

Some of these are listed in Table 10.3. The difficulties of immunising at the merozoite stage are first listed. The prospects of interfering effectively at this stage are currently not the most promising. But the door is not closed. For example, a group led by Michael Good at the Queensland Institute for Medical Research (Brisbane) and a group led by Robin Anders at the Walter and Eliza Hall Institute (Melbourne) have worked on this problem for many years and currently, clinical trials are underway in Papua New Guinea with a merozoite antigen. Robin Anders will also work with Indian scientists on malaria vaccines. Similarly, preventing or interfering with the sexual stage in mosquitoes still remains a possibility.

The finding that immunisation of experimental animals and human volunteers with x-irradiated (dead) sporozoites would protect against persistent infection by a subsequent challenge with live sporozoites was a major advance. Isolating even small numbers of sporozoites is a major task, so it is completely impractical to use such a preparation as a vaccine for whole populations. The surface antigen, the circumsporozoite (CS) protein, has been considered to be a suitable candidate as a subunit protein (it can be produced in quantity by recombinant DNA technology), but only partial protection has been achieved

Table 10.3   Difficulties versus opportunities for developing malaria vaccines

A	*The merozoite stage.*
1	RBCs are one of the few cell types that do not express major histocompatibility antigens. Specific antibody is the only immunological way to stop or interfere with the infection
2	There is considerable antigenic variation, including high mutation rates, in many important merozoite proteins
3	The proteins of interest are generally poorly immunogenic
B	*The sexual stage*
4	Theoretically, the formation of gametocyte:antibody complexes might prevent mating of gametocytes in the mosquito. This still remains an option
C	*A di- or tri-valent vaccine?*
5	Vaccinating to interfere simultaneously with two or more of the three stages of the life cycle—sporozoites, merozoites and gametocytes, is a possibility
6	A synthetic preparation (SPf166), composed of peptide sequences from three merozoite proteins and one from a sporozoite protein, has undergone clinical trials. After early limited success in some countries, later trials in the Gambia and Thailand gave very disappointing results.

in this way. Nevertheless, emphasis is shifting to preventing or curing the initial infection by sporozoites. There is an urgent need for more powerful adjuvants than the standard product, alum. This is well illustrated by a recent encouraging finding.

A hybrid preparation was made, consisting of a long peptide from the CS protein fused to a peptide from the hepatitis B virus surface antigen (HBsAg) and mixed with intact HBsAg. It was administered to human volunteers with one of three different adjuvant mixtures. Only when administered with the most complex and powerful of the three adjuvant mixtures was good protection achieved to a subsequent live sporozoite challenge. Encouragingly, protection correlated with the level of anti-CS protein antibody levels. Whether this complex adjuvant can be used safely in children remains to be seen.

Liver cells, like most mammalian cells, express class I major histocompatibility complex (MHC, or in humans, HLA antigens). The questions asked were: first, in an animal model, would transfer of CTLs clear an infection by sporozoites and so prevent the formation and release of merozoites? And secondly, could a strong CTL response be induced in humans by immunisation, and would these clear a liver infection?

Table 10.4   Findings supporting the concept that cytotoxic T lymphocytes (CTLs) could clear a sporozoite infection and so prevent the later disease

A	*Animal models.*
1	Injection of interleukin–12 (IL–12) protected monkeys against malaria. IL–12 enhances gamma interferon (IFN-γ) which in turn facilitates the maturation of CTLs
2	Immunisation of mice with a chimeric (circumsporozoite antigen, CS): adenovirus construct induced CTLs which protected against malaria disease after a sporozoite challenge
3	CS-specific CTLs could kill infected liver cells in vitro
B	*In humans*
4	The MHC class I human leucocyte antigen, Bw53, is associated with resistance to severe malaria in the Gambia. This allele is found in 15–40 per cent of the population in sub-Saharan Africa, but in less than 1 per cent of Caucasians and Asians. This suggests an evolutionary selection in Africans on the basis of protection against severe malaria

Much to the surprise of some long-time malaria investigators, the answer to the first question was 'yes'. There are reasons to believe that the answer to the second proposal might also be yes. Some are listed in Table 10.4. The association between an HLA allele and resistance to severe malaria is of particular interest as it strongly supports the development of a vaccine which induces CTL formation. Adrian Hill and colleagues (Oxford) have identified six different sporozoite proteins as sources of CTL epitopes which bind to common HLA alleles. Human volunteers will be immunised with a DNA construct followed by a chimeric poxvirus construct (see Chapter 9). The constructs may contain up to 20 different CTL epitopes identified in the six CS proteins.

Perhaps the biggest recent surprise in this area is the discovery by Geoffrey McFadden (the Botany School, University of Melbourne) that the malaria parasite contains a chloroplast, a structure which until now was considered to be present only in plants. This finding not only raises questions concerning the origin of the malaria sporozoite, but it may also open up new possibilities for the development of a better vaccine.

Developing a vaccine against *plasmodia* has proved to be quite difficult. Some years ago, the Rockefeller Foundation (New York) began a major programme on parasitic diseases. Generous financial support was given to a number of eminent medical research institutes around the world, including the Walter and Eliza Hall Institute (Melbourne). The hope was that after about a decade of intense research, vaccines would become available to control some of the diseases caused by these parasites, especially malaria. At times, over-optimistic claims were made of success being just around the corner. The task has proved to be far more difficult than was originally envisaged. After 30 or more years, and much hard work, current investigators are now more realistic in their claims. In view of our much better understanding of the infection, and increased ability to manipulate immune responses, there is reason to hope that one or more of the current efforts will prove to be successful.

CHLAMYDIA, THE TOO HIGHLY SUCCESSFUL BACTERIUM

Chlamydiae are obligate intracellular (must infect cells in order to replicate) bacteria, causing disease in humans and in animals. There are three species—*C. trachomatis, C. psittaci* and *C. pneumoniae. C. trachomatis* is strictly a human pathogen infecting primarily the genital and ocular mucosae, and causing urethritis (men), cervicitis (women) and conjunctivitis (everyone). Some infections resolve without complications but others result in serious disease. Globally, a chronic genital infection by *Chlamydia* in women causes pelvic inflammatory disease (PID), infertility and ectopic pregnancies. In the USA, chlamydia infections remain the most common treatable sexually transmitted infection, with the highest prevalence among adolescent females. The cost of diagnosis and treatment in the USA is estimated as several billion dollars per year. Recent studies have shown a greatly increased presence of *C. pneumoniae* organisms in atherosclerotic (blood vessel) lesions in cases of heart disease, compared to the near absence of these bacteria in healthy tissues.

Four different strains (serovars) of *C. trachomatis* are responsible for the disease trachoma (blindness), which occurs mainly in developing countries. Globally, it is estimated that trachoma affects about 146 million people, causes blindness in about six million, and that at least 500 million people are at serious risk of ocular infection. Repeated infections lead to blindness. Trachoma is estimated to account for 15.5 per cent of the global burden of blindness. The disease occurs where there is poverty, serious overcrowding and poor personal hygiene. In one trial (1998), children in some African villages were encouraged to wash their hands and faces at frequent intervals. It was found that 'children with sustained clean faces were much less likely to show re-emergent severe trachoma'. But this practice was unacceptable in some other villages and might be impractical in desert communities. Vaccination still offers the best hope for universal prevention.

The antibody response

The bacterium replicates in vacuoles (small, self-contained bodies surrounded by a membrane) present in the cytoplasm of mucosal cells. As bacterial antigens were not found in the rest of the cell or expressed on the plasma membrane, it was considered unlikely that infected cells would induce a cytotoxic T lymphocyte (CTL) response. Consequently, all the initial vaccine development effort was directed to inducing a strong antibody response. As well as the whole bacterium, there are two other targets. The main one is the major outer membrane protein (MOMP) at the bacterial cell surface. Its structure shows four highly variable amino acid sequences, three of which are exposed at the bacterial surface and would be recognised by antibody. The conserved sequences are hidden. The third target is a conserved (non-variable) polysaccharide molecule at the cell surface.

Though this organism is not a natural pathogen for mice (mice can clear the infection), most experiments have been done in mice. Immunisation with killed whole bacteria does not give protection and induces some ill effects. Antibody to MOMP may be protective but the great antigenic variability is the problem.

A technique called the 'anti-idiotype' approach is being used as a way to vaccinate against chlamydia. An antibody is made, part of which 'mimics' the structure of the bacterial polysaccharide model—the immune system is tricked. By immunising with this antibody, the host makes an immune response which now recognises the bacterium and prevents infection. Mice have been protected in this way from a *C. trachomatis* infection. This particular type of approach has been tried many times in other systems with little success, so there is some doubt about how effective it might be when tried in humans.

The T lymphocyte response

Both CD4+ T lymphocytes and CD8+ CTLs are induced by chlamydia infection in the mouse. A series of experiments has now shown that immunisation to induce a strong type 1 T lymphocyte response, for example, using dendritic cells exposed to dead chlamydia bacteria, gives protection. Protection is dependent upon the production of gamma interferon, which is produced by both cell types.

Again, there is a clue from the natural human infection, as was seen with both HIV and plasmodia earlier in this Chapter. A study (1998) was made of the ability of cytotoxic T lymphocytes (CTLs) in people from a trachoma-endemic region in Africa to recognise complexes between two HLA-class I molecules (B8, B35) and nonapeptides from the MOMP and from another chlamydia-specific protein. Though the number of persons investigated in this way was small (this type of investigation involves a lot of complicated laboratory work), CTLs recognising these peptide-HLA complexes were detected only in children resolving (clearing) a current infection and in adults who did not have scarring of the conjunctiva (that is, they had not suffered repeated chlamydia infections). The finding suggests that in an endemic region, the production of CTL responses during a first infection not only facilitates recovery from that infection but also helps to protect from a later infection.

The complete sequencing of the genome of *C. trachomatis* has now been achieved. It will be of great interest to see how this facilitates the development of improved vaccines. There is also increased hope that it might be possible to eliminate this disease using improved antibiotic treatment regimes. Using a combination of both approaches could be useful.

THE FUTURE

Despite the international success, especially in the twentieth century, in developing and utilising quite a large number of vaccines for infants, for adults and for the aged, there are still

Table 10.5   Some other disease agents targeted for new or improved vaccine development and for use in infants, adolescents and adults

Infants	Adolescents	Adults
Influenza (live, attenuated)	HIV–1 and 2	HIV–1 and 2
Parainfluenza	Herpes virus 2	HTLV
Respiratory syncytial virus	Gonococcus	*Helicobacter pylori*
Dengue virus	Cytomegalovirus	Staphylococcus
M. tuberculosis	*Treponema*	*M. leprae*
V. cholerae	Epstein-Barr virus	
E. coli *	Human papilloma virus	
	Hepatitis C virus	

HIV = human immunodeficiency virus; HTLV = human T-cell lymphotrophic virus.
*   Especially those strains secreting strong toxins (enterotoxigenic, ETEC) and causing haemorrhages (enterihaemorrhagic, EHEC).

a number of very serious infections where availability of an effective vaccine would be a great boon to society in general. Steady progress is being made for some of these. For example, the first rotavirus and Lyme disease (*Borrelia burgdorferi*) vaccines have recently been licensed in the USA. Table 10.5 lists some other diseases where vaccines are urgently needed. There are a number of other infections, such as Ebola virus, where the infection, though usually fatal, is confined to such a small region that the expense of vaccine development may not be justified.

We hope that the three diseases reviewed in this Chapter will illustrate to the reader that developing a vaccine is not always straightforward. In the case of an infectious agent (plasmodia) that may have evolved with humans over a long period, it can be a difficult, time-consuming and expensive task. Plasmodia have adjusted their pattern of infection and reproduction to evade the human immune response. On the other hand, HIV is an example of how rapidly a new infectious agent with a RNA genome, which allows rapid mutations to occur, can adjust from one host, the chimpanzee, to another, humans. The slaughter of very large numbers of chickens has been the only way to deal with suddenly emerging new strains of bird influenza, another RNA virus.

For the three diseases discussed in this Chapter, there is now hope that a new approach to vaccine development, based primarily on inducing a type 1 T cell response, may be more successful than approaches based solely on an antibody response. In each case, possession of certain class I HLA alleles (specificities) which correlate with protection from severe disease in endemic areas has given scientists an important clue on how to proceed further with vaccine development.

11

The potential for the control of non-communicable diseases by vaccination or immunotherapy

This chapter reports on progress being made to control three different situations: two types of non-communicable disease—autoimmunity (immune responses against the body) and neoplasia (cancer)—and attempts to control fertility. Though very few of the procedures to be described have yet been licensed for general human use, the results from model systems are encouraging and many clinical trials are underway.

The technical background for the work described in this chapter was presented in Chapters 4 and 5.

Part 1—Immunotherapy to control autoimmune diseases

Currently, autoimmune diseases—the immune system reacting against self antigens—are controlled by drugs which suppress the immune system as a whole. Though useful, this is a very non-selective approach. In the last few decades, there have been extensive studies aimed at understanding the precise nature of some of the more common diseases—which host antigens are targeted by antibodies or T cells, whether an infectious agent is involved and whether there are particular human leucocyte antigen (HLA, or MHC) associations. A number of diseases are associated with particular HLA alleles, the most striking being ankylosing spondylitis, where there is an 85 per cent association with HLA B27. The symptoms of ankylosing spondylitis are great stiffness and curvature of the spine. There are a number of autoimmune diseases about which comparatively little is known, but Table 11.1 describes some of the known and possible associations in the case of the more common autoimmune diseases.

Autoimmune diseases can occur because of cross-reactivity between an infectious agent and a host cell antigen, for example, an antibody made against the infectious agent also reacts with a normal host component. A well-studied example is rheumatic fever in which antibodies to the cell wall of the streptococcus bacterium cross-react with cardiac muscle protein. In this case, it should be possible to make a bacterial protein vaccine in which the amino acid sequence which mimics the muscle protein has been excised. This vaccine could be used to immunise people against this bacterial infection and so prevent rheumatic fever.

In several other experimental situations, the evidence is now very strong that activated T lymphocytes cause the disease. Administration of specific T lymphocytes in animal models has induced the symptoms of autoimmune diseases, including arthritis, thyroiditis, insulin-dependent diabetes mellitus (IDDM) and systemic lupus erythematosus (SLE). In the case of experimental autoimmune encephalomyelitis (EAE), a widely used model for multiple sclerosis (MS) in humans, administration of T cells specific for the brain protein, myelin, causes the disease. Furthermore, and not unexpectedly, it is the type 1 T lymphocyte (CD4+) which is responsible.

What are the possible immunological approaches to preventing (prophylaxis) or modifying (immunotherapy) the course of these diseases?

There are a surprising number of approaches which have been or are under investigation. Five 'mainstream' ones are as follows:

Table 11.1   Common autoimmune diseases; the mechanism involved, antigens recognised and possible association with different infections

Disease	Causal mechanism	Known or possible infection	Antigen recognised
Rheumatic fever	antibody	Streptococcus	Cardiac muscle
Systemic lupus erythematosis	antibody	A retrovirus	DNA
Insulin-dependent diabetes mellitus	T cells	Coxsackie virus?	Antigens in the pancreas*
Experimental autoimmune encephalomyelitis**	T cells		Myelin basic protein
Multiple sclerosis	T cells	?	?
Rheumatoid arthritis	T cells	Epstein-Barr virus	Synovial joint antigens
Hashimoto's thyroiditis	T cells	Mumps virus?	Thyroid hormone

*   Including insulin and two enzymes.

**   Experimental autoimmune encephalomyelitis (EAE) is a convenient model for multiple sclerosis.

APPROACHES TO PREVENT OR MODIFY THE PROGRESS OF AUTOIMMUNE DISEASES IN EXPERIMENTAL MODELS

1   immunising with inactivated, CD4+ T lymphocytes which are highly specific for the target host antigen—this approach is sometimes called T-cell vaccination;

2   identification of the dominant cytokine(s) produced by the activated type 1 CD4+ T lymphocytes, and neutralisation of its (their) activity by specific antibody;

3   switching the type 1 T lymphocyte response to a type 2 response by the introduction of specific cytokines, or by neutralising the role of the cytokine IL–12 which favours a type 1 response (Chapter 4);

4   immunising with the specific target antigen (when known) under conditions which favour a type 2 T lymphocyte response; and

5   inducing a state of immunological tolerance to the target antigen.

Though some progress is being made in each of these approaches, two (numbers 2 and 5) are further advanced or seem more promising, and are now discussed in more detail.

Treatment of those with rheumatoid arthritis to alleviate the disease-inducing effect of a dominant cytokine

Type 1 CD4+ T lymphocytes which mediate arthritis secrete a number of different cytokines, some of which contribute to inflammation in the bone joints by activating a variety of different cell types which invade the joint. Careful study has shown that of the different cytokines produced by these type 1 lymphocytes, one, called the tumour necrosis factor alpha (TNFα), is primarily responsible for activating the invading cells, such as macrophages. The concept arose by asking—would it be possible to make a strong antibody which would bind to and so 'neutralise' the activity of the TNFα? (approach (2) as described above). By regular passive transfer of such an antibody preparation, the painful effects of arthritis would be overcome. The preparation made is called a monoclonal antibody because every antibody molecule has the same antigen-binding specificity, so that it should be a very effective preparation. Such preparations are easily made in mouse cells, but not in human cells. But if mouse antibody was to be regularly transfused into humans, it would be recognised as foreign, and destroyed by the human immune system. The ameliorating effect of transfusion would be very short-lived. So Marc Feldmann and his colleagues in London, who have worked on this approach for many years, made a chimeric antibody—part mouse and part human amino acid sequences (the mouse antibody was 'humanised'). This preparation has been well tolerated in patients and has so successfully (to date) tricked the human immune system that it has been possible to regularly transfuse the preparation into humans.

This preparation was approved by the FDA in 1998 for use in the USA in treating rheumatoid arthritis patients. It is not yet clear whether it can be given indefinitely.

Induction of a state of tolerance to antigens recognised in autoimmune disease

It will be recalled (Chapter 9) that following oral administration of a soluble foreign protein, a state of tolerance ensued. Thus, if the host was subsequently challenged systemically by the same antigen, a very weak response compared to that of controls was observed. That is, the tolerance achieved was substantial but not complete. Studies showed that the tolerance was at the level of T cell responses, and did not directly affect B cells, except that T cell-dependent B cell responses were greatly reduced. The question arose—if a soluble preparation of the target antigen was fed orally, would it mitigate the expression of disease in those cases where autoimmune disease occurred which was mediated by Th1 T cells?

It was found that oral administration of a target antigen such as myelin basic protein (MPB) to mice induced a Th 2 response and this has been a general but not an absolutely universal finding. Several clinical trials have been performed or are underway using this approach to treat patients with auto-immune diseases such as multiple sclerosis or arthritis. The trials were double blind and with placebo controls (only half the group receive the active drug, but neither doctor nor patients know whether a patient is receiving active drug or inactive placebo until the end of the trial). Sometimes, the placebo group has done surprisingly well, and if this happens, it is more difficult to interpret the overall results. Phase II and III clinical trials have been and are being carried out with oral doses of a collagen preparation (collagen is a major bone protein) to establish whether the effects of arthritis can be mitigated. The results to date are rather borderline with no success in some trials and partial success in others. Some studies are continuing.

Meanwhile, a completely unexpected observation led to quite a different focus for research.

Minimising the proliferation of autoreactive T lymphocytes

In 1968, Brian Greenwood (from the UK but based in Gambia, Africa) noted that although there was a very low occurrence of autoimmune diseases in tropical Africa, Africans born and resident in a non-tropical, developed country could have high levels of autoimmune diseases. Obviously, the effect was not primarily genetically based but had to be largely an environmental effect. He proposed that the difference was caused by the exposure, since childhood, of Africans living in tropical Africa to multiple parasitic infections. This can lead to adult

Africans being permanently parasitised by malaria but showing few symptoms—they not only appear to be 'tolerant' to malaria, but they also become immunosuppressed (respond poorly to other infections or vaccines). A group at the John Curtin School in Canberra, led by Ian Clark and Bill Cowden, followed this up and found that people infected with malaria and/or other parasites had very high levels of nitric oxide in their macrophages and this inhibited T cell responses. They proposed that Africans born in Africa have naturally (through evolutionary pressures) low levels of nitric oxide in their macrophages so that the build-up of nitric oxide following exposure to multiple parasites would not be quite so drastic. It was argued that, if born in and resident in a developed country where exposure to several parasites would be very rare, their inherent low level of nitric oxide made those of African descent able to make strong immune responses but this may include an increased susceptibility to some autoimmune diseases.

With David Willenborg, they tested their ideas in two opposite ways. A strain of rats, PVG, is normally very resistant to developing experimental autoimmune encephalomyelitis (EAE, the animal model corresponding to human multiple sclerosis) when immunised with the target antigen. There are relatively high levels of nitric oxide in their cells. Following treatment with a chemical which *specifically* lowers nitric oxide levels, and then immunising with the target antigen (myelin protein), EAE was found to occur much more frequently in the treated compared to untreated rats. As a complete contrast, the question was then asked—was it possible to increase nitric oxide levels in an animal model and so decrease the rate of the *natural* occurrence of an autoimmune disease? Fortunately, there is a strain of mice, the NOD (non-obese, diabetic) mice, of which a high proportion spontaneously develop diabetes, like some people. These mice have been immunised in different ways and the incidence of diabetes decreased. Recently, this group found that immunisation enhanced nitric oxide levels and this increase coincided with the treated mice failing to develop diabetes.

Greatly encouraged by these results, the group has joined forces with Kevin Lafferty (Director, John Curtin School, 1993–8) who has had a long-time interest in human diabetes. In phase I clinical trials, one group of subjects who have a disposition to develop diabetes will be immunised with a registered human vaccine which should mimic some of the effects of a parasitic infection, and cause an increase in nitric oxide levels. The group will then be monitored and compared with the incidence of diabetes in a control, non-immunised group.

PROSPECTS

There is now a good deal of optimism that by using one or preferentially a combination of these approaches, it should be possible to help those who are susceptible to or suffer from autoimmune diseases. It may be that one particular approach will be found to be more effective for one or other disease. In some cases where there is a significant HLA association, it may be possible to prevent the development of a particular auto-immune disease. Probably more generally, the aim would be to mitigate substantially the pathological effects of the particular disease, especially if people could be diagnosed very early in the development of the disease.

Part 2—Immunotherapy to control/cure cancers

The attempt to develop cancer vaccines was based initially on the concept that there were immunological differences between normal cells and cancer cells. Two very eminent scientists, Lewis Thomas (USA) and Macfarlane Burnet (Melbourne) proposed in the late 1950s that tumours were normally prevented from occurring because they were recognised by the immune system as being 'different' to normal cells, and were destroyed. Burnet coined the term—'immunosurveillance' to describe the process. It has been known for some time that a few tumours, especially melanomas, may spontaneously regress, and in several cases, it has now been established that this regression is due to mutations which have made that particular tumour highly susceptible to destruction by cytotoxic T lymphocytes. However, this regression is the exception rather than the rule.

The great majority of tumours progress because they manage to evade the immune system. Most tumours occur in people with no apparent immunodeficiency. Children and mice born *without* an effective adaptive immune system (*severe* combined immunodeficient, called for short SCID) have a higher rate of malignancy than 'normal' children or mice, but the incidence is still quite low because they have relatively short lives. The laboratory-bred SCID mice *mimic* a very small proportion of children who are *not* normal but are born with this severe deficiency. Unless they live in a 'special suit' designed to prevent exposure to infections, they soon die.

Frequently, initial small foci of cancer cells are kept under control by other non-immune mechanisms. When these other mechanisms break down, a tumour can grow in an uncontrolled fashion. That is, the tumour progresses beyond this initial stage because it evades the immune system. The legacy of Thomas and of Burnet was the stimulation of much research that has led to the present level of understanding. A brief summary follows:

1 Some viral infections may lead to tumours in a proportion of those infected. These cancer cells will express one or more antigens of the infecting virus.
2 The majority of tumours are not associated with viral infections. They may express antigens which are a modified form of an antigen expressed on other normal cell types in the body; or the antigens are expressed in greater quantity compared to the level on one or more different types of normal cells.
3 Tumours progress and cause death because they either evade or 'de-rail' the immune response.

VIRUSES AND CANCER

Viral infections are involved in about 15 per cent of all human cancers and Table 11. 2 lists the major contributors. The first three in the table are of major significance. There are two major questions: first, if people are vaccinated against the responsible virus before cancer formation is initiated, will the tumour no longer occur? and second, if the tumour expresses viral antigens, why are these not recognised by the immune system? We are beginning to find the answers to both of these questions.

Table 11.2   Viral infections associated with human cancers

Virus	Type of cancer
Hepatitis viruses, especially hepatitis B	Liver cancer
HIV–1	Kaposi's sarcoma
	B-cell lymphomas
Papilloma (HPV16, HPV18*)	Genital carcinoma
Papilloma (HPV5, HPV8*)	Squamous cell carcinoma
Epstein-Barr	Burkitt's lymphoma
	Nasopharyngeal carcinoma
HTLV–1,2**	Adult T cell leukaemia

*   Viral types most commonly involved; HPV, human papilloma virus.
**   Human T cell leukaemia viruses.

Hepatitis B and liver cancer

Hepatitis B virus can be transmitted from mother to baby at birth or acquired later in life through sexual intercourse, intravenous injection, etc. The highest incidence of infection occurs in China (about 10 per cent) compared to 0.1 per cent in the USA. Japan has the highest incidence of any industrialised country. At any one time, there are at least several hundred million carriers of hepatitis B virus infections worldwide, mainly in Asia and in equatorial Africa. There are 68 million new cases in the world each year and about 600,000 deaths (Table 11.3). Although most cases of liver cancer caused by hepatitis B virus infection occur between ages 30–50, they do occur but less frequently in childhood. Integration of the viral DNA into the genome of the host liver cell is considered to be a pre-requisite for cancer to develop.

Late last century, a German scientist Robert Koch postulated the types of information needed to be acquired in order to prove that a particular disease agent caused a certain disease; they are known as Koch's Postulates. Koch was concerned mainly with infections in animal models, and the major postulate was that administration of the infectious agent to the animal host should cause the disease. However, there is no suitable animal model for many infectious agents. In such situations, the most direct way would be to deliberately infect a person with the agent and to show that the disease then occurs. In the great majority of cases, it would be completely unethical to do this. Another direct method would be to show that if that particular naturally occurring infection could be *specifically* prevented, the disease would not occur. Once a hepatitis B viral vaccine became available, this second approach became possible.

In mid-1984, a nationwide hepatitis B vaccination programme was implemented in Taiwan where, like China, the prevalence of this infection is very high. By 1997, the following data on the incidence of liver cancer and of deaths from this cancer in children, expressed per 100,000 were:

(i) liver cancer incidence, 6–14-year-old children,
    1981–6, 0.7; 1986–90, 0.57; 1990–4, 0.36:
(ii) liver cancer deaths, 6–9-year-old children,
    born between 1974 and 1984, 0.52;
    born between 1984 and 1986, 0.13.

As a control, the incidence of brain tumours in children 6–14 years of age was shown not to decline during this period.

These differences in the liver cancer results are highly significant. While findings with older vaccinated individuals are awaited with great interest, the present results are highly encouraging and go very close to fulfilling the postulate outlined above. Furthermore, it is the first time that a specific immunological treatment has reduced the incidence of deaths from cancer in more than 50 per cent of a cohort (a like group) of individuals. A similar trial is being carried out in Gambia by the International Agency for Research on Cancer, but has not been in progress for long enough to obtain a clear-cut result.

Papilloma virus and genital cancer

Papilloma viruses have a DNA genome and cause lesions in the epithelial cells of humans and animals. There are well over 100 different strains of the virus and infection by some of these is closely associated with the occurrence of different cancers. Cervical cancer is the best studied because it occurs worldwide. Eighty per cent of cervical cancers are associated with one of four human papilloma virus (HPV) types, and mainly with HPV16. It is now generally accepted that HPV infection is a pre-requisite for the development of nearly all cases of cervical carcinoma. There is a lower level of association of HPV types with other cancers such as those involving the penis, anus and vagina, and with genital warts. Worldwide, these cancers afflict nearly half a million women and 100,000 men. Cervical cancer is predicted to result in about 200,000 deaths worldwide in 1999. However, a surprisingly large number of women in the world, estimates run as high as 300 million, are carriers of HPV DNA but exhibit no clinical symptoms.

As with hepatitis B virus, the emphasis is on developing a prophylactic vaccine against HPV infection, and here the prospect is encouraging. There is no attempt to develop a live attenuated viral vaccine because of the potential danger that it might cause cancer. Instead, the aim is to develop a subunit vaccine. Ian Frazer at the University of Queensland is working on this approach. The principal antigen of the viral 'coat' is the protein, L1, which when isolated, can re-assemble to form a mosaic of units, forming structures called virus-like particles (VLPs). Immunising dogs, rabbits and even cattle with the L1 VLPs prepared from the corresponding specific papilloma viruses induces antibodies which protect against a challenge infection. The protective role of antibody is confirmed by transfusing the isolated antibody to naive (uninfected) hosts before challenge. Importantly, this viral infectivity-neutralising antibody recognises a 'conformational' epitope caused by the association of the L1 molecules. It binds poorly to individual L1 molecules. This effect is also seen with other viruses (see also Chapters 2 and 10). Three phase I clinical trials of these VLPs are, at time of writing, close to conclusion, with encouragingly high titres (levels of activity) of antibodies being formed.

Therefore, the current indications are that HPV vaccines can be developed which have the potential to inhibit HPV infection and hence prevent the establishment of these tumours. As with the occurrence of liver cancer following hepatitis B virus infection, it will take many years to show whether such an immunisation schedule will largely if not completely prevent the development of cervical cancer in women. But because this cancer can occur to a lesser extent in young women, a period of about ten years after initiating a programme to immunise young adolescents might be sufficient to indicate a significant protective effect, as was the case following immunisation with hepatitis B virus. It will also be of great interest to see whether the incidence of the other cancers mentioned above can also be reduced in this way.

Immunotherapy for cervical cancer

In view of the high prevalence of and mortality due to cervical cancer, there is an equally pressing need to develop an immunotherapeutic approach especially for the control and hopefully resolution of this cancer. Papilloma viruses contain an oncogene (a gene which following infection, is inserted into the host cell genome and induces cancer development). The protein product of this gene, E7, is the prime target for an immunological attack. Ian Frazer and his colleagues at the University of Queensland have purified this protein and have shown that when mice were immunised with it, they resisted a challenge with HPV 16 tumour cells. This protein product is currently being tested in a clinical trial.

HIV and cancer

Prior to the AIDS epidemic, Kaposi's sarcoma (KS) was a rare tumour except in a few regions of the world. As the prevalence of AIDS increased, KS was reported in 20–50 per cent of AIDS patients, a very large increase in cancer incidence, though this level may have decreased in recent years. The effect of the HIV infection may be indirect, being due to high levels of certain cytokines produced during the infection, and superinfection of HIV patients by another virus, human herpes virus 8.

B lymphocyte lymphoma is also now found more commonly in HIV-infected individuals as they progress towards AIDS. There is a variety of other tumours which may be associated with the development of AIDS, but the available information is insufficient to ascribe HIV infection as being the cause.

As with the other tumours, the widespread use of an effective prophylactic HIV vaccine will be a deciding factor in elucidating the role of HIV in the occurrence of these tumours (Chapter 10). In the meantime, there is encouraging evidence that in mice, generation of a strong CD8+ T lymphocyte response can eradicate a B-lymphoma and protect against a later challenge.

PROSPECTS

All the viruses mentioned in Table 11.2 are targets for vaccine development. In the long term, the aim would be to immunise those known to be at risk of infection by these viruses prior to that risk occurring—mainly before adolescence in the case of sexually transmitted diseases (STDs). It is not unreasonable to believe that in due course (10–15 years time), programmes will be in place to achieve such an outcome, along the lines of the current hepatitis B vaccination programme in Taiwan. In the interim, it may prove possible to cause the regression of some of these tumours by vaccination. Tumours caused by papilloma viruses are a good example.

OTHER CANCERS

Most cancers arise independently of any infectious agent, and for some years now the search has been on to identify any antigens expressed by the cell which are largely or completely unique to the tumour. It is now known that many tumours express antigens which are either in greater quantity than found on normal cells, or which differ qualitatively from those expressed on normal cells.

Mainly, two immunological approaches for immunotherapy to control/clear the tumour are being investigated—the use of highly specific antibodies and the generation of cytotoxic T lymphocyte (CTL) responses or, if feasible, the induction of both responses.

Antibody-based immunotherapy

The ability to generate in large quantity highly specific antibodies, called monoclonal antibodies (meaning all molecules have the same specificity) has been a great advance. Such antibodies with a very high specificity for tumour antigens are being used in several ways:

- the antibody is made highly radioactive, so that when it binds to the target tumour cell, the radioactivity will harm the cell and prevent it growing further;
- a cellular poison is attached to the antibody. The role of the antibody then is to deliver the poison to the targeted cell and this can lead to the death of the tumour cell;
- the antibodies can be modified so that instead of poison, they transport cytokines or even CTLs to the tumour. This is a way to directly facilitate the interaction of these products with the tumour cells.

188

With the exception of transporting CTLs to the tumour, these approaches have the great advantage that the antibody should be effective when administered to anybody with that particular tumour, independent of the genetic make-up of the individual.

The first two approaches work very well in the test tube but when used in vivo (in the body), there have been difficulties. One is that some of the preparations can non-specifically bind to other cells and this can cause toxicity, especially to the liver. Another is that because these antibodies are made in mice, they have to be 'humanised' in order not to be rejected by the human host if given repeatedly. A third is that the antigen(s) must be expressed at the tumour cell surface for it to be seen by the antibody. Fourthly, the target antigen may mutate, so that it is no longer recognised by the antibody. Nevertheless, some clinical trials are underway to test the efficiency of this approach with particular tumours, such as lymphomas.

Sometimes, tumour cells express unique carbohydrates at their surface, and this is the case with prostate cancer cells. A cluster of such molecules has now been synthesised and conjugated to protein to enhance their ability to induce a strong antibody response when they are used to immunise cancer patients. Clinical trials are underway on patients who have undergone prostate surgery (removal of the prostate) to see whether recurrences of the cancer can be prevented.

Melanomas express compounds called glycolipids (combinations of sugars and fats) at their surface. One member, GM2, of a group called gangliosides has been conjugated to a protein and, with an adjuvant called QS–21, is being administered to melanoma patients in a phase III clinical trial. This is the final assessment of a vaccine for safety and efficacy, before it can be approved for general use to treat melanoma patients.

Immunotherapy involving the generation of CTLs

This has become the most popular approach, mainly because the cytotoxic T lymphocytes (CTLs) should recognise *any* tumour-specific protein antigen which was not present before birth, that is, to which the host is not tolerant. Furthermore, the spontaneous regresson of some melanomas has now been shown to be due to CTLs recognising a peptide epitope which has mutated and is now recognised better by the immune system. In addition, the results with model systems have been very encouraging. Using tumours which grow in mice, it has been possible to immunise the mice to induce CTLs specific for a tumour antigen. Transfer of the tumour to these immunised mice has frequently resulted in the prevention of tumour growth, and transfer of such CTLs to mice with an already established tumour has sometimes resulted in complete regression of the tumour.

With such encouraging results, there has been an intensive search for human tumour antigens which could be targets for CTLs. Table 11.3 lists some of the tumours examined. The aim has been twofold: first, to examine the level of specificity of an antigen for the particular tumour, and second, to see whether there are several antigens which are reasonably specific for each type of tumour. The reason for this second point is the possibility that one or two antigens alone might not contain CTL epitopes which would be well recognised by the CD8+ T lymphocytes (precursors of CTLs) of a wide variety of people. The net result is that for some tumours, several such antigens have been identified. The record is probably held by melanomas where more than a dozen antigens have now been described. Furthermore, some of these antigens are also present on other tumour cells. Generally, they have not been found on normal cells or in tissues, exceptions being melanocytes and testicular cells in the case of some melanoma antigens.

There are several factors which make the task of a tumour vaccine more difficult than vaccinating to prevent a subsequent acute viral infection:

1 The target antigen may be subject to mutation, and so escapes an already established immune response. The ex-pression of class I MHC antigen at the cancer cell surface may be greatly reduced, so that the tumour can then evade a CTL response as it is no longer recognised by these cells.
2 Cells of some tumours can secrete products which harm and inactivate CTLs, but ways are being explored to overcome this problem.

Table 11.3 Tumours examined for antigens which could be targets for cytotoxic T lymphocyte attack

Carcinomas
Bladder, mammary (breast), head and neck squamous cell, non-small cell lung, colorectal, rectal

Others
Melanomas, leukaemias, lymphomas

3   To expand, tumours need to develop a blood supply system, including capillary vessels. These can be defective in such a way that although the tumour can grow, access to the tumour cells by immune cells such as CTLs can be restricted.

Though they express novel antigens, tumour cells obviously don't act as antigen-presenting cells (APCs) and so induce an immune response (which could destroy them). To change this, one approach has been to 'convert' them to APCs by 'transfecting' them with DNA coding for certain cytokines such as GM-CSF (granulocyte macrophage colony stimulating factor). In addition, this attracts 'professional' APCs, dendritic cells, into the tumour and thus increases the chance of an effective immune response against the tumour being initiated. In model systems, this approach has been fairly successful.

Extraction of the cells comprising a tumour mass has shown in many cases that the mixture contains TILs—tumour infiltrating lymphocytes, including CD8+ T cells, which are ready to be activated. Alternatively, these TILs can be removed, cultivated in vitro with other cytokines such as interleukin–2 (IL–2) to activate them and then re-administered. This has resulted in regression of the tumour in some cases.

With the continuing identification of new tumour-specific antigens, it has been possible to identify peptide epitopes (nonamers) which would bind to certain major histocompatibility antigen alleles (specificities, see Table 4.3), such as HLA–A1. When such peptides from the tumour antigen, MAGE–3, were administered to 25 patients with metastatic (i.e., growing at multiple sites in the body) melanoma and possessing the HLA–A1 specificity, there were three complete remissions (cure) and four partial remissions. In another trial involving 36 HLA–A2 melanoma patients given cancer antigen peptides and GM-CSF, 25 patients were evaluated. Four responded clinically and 11 showed stabilisation of the disease. In another similar trial, 13 out of 31 patients with metastatic melanoma and possessing the HLA–A2 allele and who were immunised with a synthetic peptide vaccine with interleukin–2, responded positively. Tumour regression occurred in skin, lymph nodes, lung, and notably in the liver and brain, regions where in previous attempts, it had been difficult to clear tumours. These results are particularly encouraging.

Another related approach is to first generate a patient's dendritic cells (DCs) by culturing precursor cells present in the blood and then to pulse (treat for short periods) them with tumour antigen peptides, with the whole tumour antigen or with complete tumour cell extracts. The treated DCs are then administered to the patients. The highly successful animal experiments reported earlier used this approach. In one clinical trial, 16 patients with advanced melanoma were immunised with their own (mainly peptide) pulsed DCs and five showed improvement with regression of metastases in various organs.

Though melanomas have become the favoured tumour for these investigations, similar studies are in progress with other human tumours. Breast carcinoma cells express a glycoprotein (protein with sugar side chains) called MUC1. It differs in several respects from the glycoprotein expressed on normal cells. Ian McKenzie and colleagues at the Austin Research Institute (Melbourne) are developing an immunotherapeutic approach based on generating CTLs specific for MUC1. The patient's cultured DCs are pulsed with MUC1 and then administered back to the patient. Clinical trials are currently underway.

THE OUTLOOK FOR THE FUTURE

Though it is best to be cautious about future prospects, it is difficult not to express a degree of optimism about the pace of progress in this area of cancer immunotherapy. Barely more than a decade ago, the approaches to cancer immunotherapy were a shadow of today's sophisticated investigations. And the way forward from current work seems reasonably clear.

The aim is to identify several antigens specific for the cancer so the appoach to treatment is multi-antigen specific. Though mutations occur fairly readily, they are unlikely to occur at the same time in all antigens. (This is a similar argument to that used for multi-drug therapy of infections like HIV.) Furthermore, if a CTL response is to be used, this offers a wider range of peptide epitopes to which most in a population could respond.

Initial clinical trials are usually performed with patients whose disease is well advanced. Once a technique is shown to be safe and reasonably effective in such a trial, it can be applied to patients at a much earlier stage of disease, or after major surgery to remove most of the tumour, for example after removal of a tumour of the prostate or breast.

It may of course turn out that, even as present approaches are refined and improved, the success rate may never quite reach the 80–90 per cent level. The final solution to curing many cancers could involve a combination therapy. One possibility would be an immune-based immunisation protocol together with one of the new approaches to prevent angiogenesis—the formation of new blood vessels upon which growth of a solid tumour is absolutely dependent. Recent advances in this field have also been spectacular, at least in model systems.

Part 3—Vaccines to control human fertility

Despite the fact that sexual reproduction in mammals is a relatively inefficient process (Chapter 9), requiring the production of huge numbers of sperm, the main danger to the planet Earth is overpopulation by humans. The population is increasing at the rate of about 1 billion each decade which could lead to disastrous social and environmental consequences. This increase is occurring mainly in developing countries where the current technologies used in developed countries to control fertility are less available or the people are discouraged from using them.

Is there a need for an additional method of fertility control to be available in such situations? In the early 1970s, the Human Reproduction Programme (HRP) of the WHO thought so and established a Task Force to report on immunological methods for fertility regulation, and especially on the safety and efficacy of using self or self-like antigens as the basis of the vaccine. This resulted in the formation of a vaccine unit within the HRP which operated for about 20 years.

SAFETY REQUIREMENTS FOR A HUMAN FERTILITY CONTROL VACCINE

There already was evidence that immunological reactions against self could interfere with human reproduction. Some women make anti-sperm antibodies and become infertile (Chapter 9). Different cytokines, notably IL1α, TNFα and IFNγ can inhibit oestrogen production and normal follicle development.

In the late 1970s, general guidelines for a human fertility control vaccine were established by the WHO. They included:

1 the target antigen should be essential for the reproductive process;
2 to minimise the risk of autoimmune disease, the target antigen should be specific to the reproductive process;
3 as a further safeguard, the target antigen should occur only at a critical stage of the reproductive process; and
4 the effects of vaccination should be reversible after a given period (1–2 years) following which an immunised woman should be able to initiate a normal pregnancy resulting in a healthy child.

POTENTIAL TARGET ANTIGENS

The target antigens are mainly of two types: hormones of the conceptus (the fertilised egg prior to implantation) (and the main emphasis has been on the human chorionic gonadotrophin hormone, hCG) ; and gamete antigens (antigens of the sperm or egg).

Human chorionic gonadotrophin as a target antigen

Though trace amounts of human chorionic gonadotrophin (hCG) occur in non-pregnant women, hCG production is greatly boosted once fertilisation of the egg occurs. High concentrations are necessary for implantation of the conceptus in the uterus to occur, and in the maintenance of early pregnancy. The presence of high levels of hCG is widely used to diagnose pregnancy. This hormone contains an α and β polypeptide chain. The same α chain is present in three other hormones produced in the pituitary gland so that attention has been mainly focused on the β chain which is 145 amino acids long. The final (C-terminal end) 37 amino acid sequence does not show any cross-reactivity with other hormones.

Two approaches have been made:

1   The approach mainly supported by the HRP/WHO vaccine unit was based on a conjugate of the 37 amino acid C-terminal peptide of βhCG with diphtheria toxoid. It was administered with particular adjuvants and was first submitted to exhaustive trials in other primates. It underwent a phase I clinical trial in sterile women. Though completely specific, the antibody response to this preparation was reported by others to be less than ideal.

2   The approach supported by the Indian Council for Medical Research and under the direction of Pran Talwar was based on a preparation containing the complete βhCG subunit. When linked to the α chain of the luteinising hormone (LH), and conjugated to diphtheria or to tetanus toxoids, higher levels of anti-βhCG antibody were produced. The two preparations were administered sequentially and with adjuvant. This vaccine has been used in a phase II clinical trial with women of reproductive age who were known to be fertile (already had children), had an active sexual life and normal ovulatory cycles. Collectively, 1227 menstrual cycles were recorded during the trial, and only one pregnancy occurred. The level of the anti-hCG antibodies produced correlated with their ability to neutralise the activity of hCG. In practice, it would be necessary to monitor anti-hCG antibody levels at set intervals to know when to re-immunise, if continued contraception was desired.

Targeting gamete antigens

A variety of sperm antigens have been described and some isolated and studied. Some such as lactate dehydrogenase and fertilisation antigen, have been studied in detail and antibodies raised against them have prevented conception to various extents in animal models, mainly rodents, guinea pigs and rabbits.

The mammalian oocyte (egg) is surrounded by a translucent matrix called the zona pellucida (ZP) which the sperm must penetrate in order to fertilise the egg. The ZP contains three glycoproteins (proteins with side-chains composed of different sugars)—ZP1, ZP2 and ZP3. From studies in different animals, especially the pig, ZP3 seems to be the important target for sperm to engage in order to effect entry into the egg itself.

There is considerable interest in using vaccination to control fertility in animal populations, rather than control by killing. This has been achieved in the USA with a population of wild horses on the Assateague island off the coast of South Carolina. In Australia, there is a major project (a Co-operative Research Centre) to see whether populations of pests such as rabbits, foxes and mice can be controlled in this way, rather than by poisoning or shooting. In this project, chimeric live vectors, such as certain viruses, would be used to deliver the vaccine antigens to the host population.

PROSPECTS

The results of the Indian trial look promising but the test will come when this or similar preparations are used on a much larger scale, in the long run possibly by millions rather than scores of women. If autoimmunity, especially against the LH component of the candidate vaccine, does not occur, it should prove to be a worthwhile addition to other fertility control techniques, especially in a country such as India.

Epilogue

In developing countries, immunisations are recognised as being enormously important. In developed countries, in contrast, the common attitude observed is complacency. Once smallpox began to disappear in developed countries in the nineteenth century, there was a tendency to think that the infection had been conquered and that continuing vaccination with its unpleasant side reactions was unnecessary. It needed the continuing presence of sick or dying naturally infected individuals to convince many of the crucial role of vaccination. Close to the twenty-first century, with so many childhood infections reduced to very low levels largely by vaccination, the same complacency occurs. This is enhanced by the fact that most children infected by these agents undergo a subclinical infection, that is, they appear not to be affected by the infection. Fortunately, most parents accept the advice of their health provider, but some are swayed by the arguments of those in the anti-vaccination lobby.

We have presented data showing that present-day vaccines are effective, but some are better than others. With very few exceptions, the data show that the vaccines are very safe, especially when compared to the level of early side effects or delayed adverse reactions following the natural infection. However, if a scientifically valid association between vaccination and a serious adverse effect can be demonstrated, there should be a mechanism for compensation.

We have stressed several aspects which are not widely appreciated. The efficacy of a vaccine depends upon the immune response that it induces. This response is genetically determined and apart from identical twins, virtually everybody has a unique combination of the genes which determine the immune response. This means that all of us will have different patterns of response to a wide variety of infectious diseases and to the corresponding vaccines. Most individuals will respond well to most vaccines; the vaccines would not be licensed for human use if this was not the case. Many individuals may respond poorly to one or a few vaccines (a different pattern for each individual), so that in these latter cases, they may become sick if later exposed to the natural infection. For this reason, such individuals are often called non-responders to that vaccine. This implies that the vaccine is inefficient. This could apply more to subunit vaccines such as the hepatitis B vaccine. But it is more likely that the individual lacks genes which would allow a stronger response to that particular vaccine. The general experience is that in such cases, the illness so experienced will be much less severe and life-threatening compared to the effect if the child had not been pre-vaccinated. An immunological explanation for this effect is that, even though a child may show a very low specific antibody response to a given vaccine, the overall response is sufficient to 'prime' the immune system. This results in a more rapid immune response to the later infection, resulting in partial protection from disease.

With very few exceptions, the susceptibility of a child to serious disease and possibly death by a particular infection, say measles, cannot yet be predicted. In the absence of this information, the safest procedure by far is to immunise the child. Being healthy per se does not confer protection.

The data in Table 5.1 should convince everyone about the efficacy of the childhood vaccines, including one of the latest, the Hib vaccine. Contrast this data with the incidence in the 1990s of two other childhood diseases, caused by rotavirus and respiratory syncytial virus, for which at that time, no vaccines were available. With rotavirus infections, the incidence of disease in the USA and in developing countries is almost identical.

In a recent edition of the Children's Vaccine Initiative (CVI)

Forum (17, November 1998), an article, 'Vaccination—now the right of all children', discusses the right of children to be vaccinated. The authors state: 'In fact, vaccination is a right, enshrined by implication or explicitly in at least eight legally binding international instruments'. Of these, the Convention on the Rights of the Child, adopted by the UN General Assembly in November, 1989, has been the most widely accepted (191 countries by 1998). The situation might be interpreted as follows.

If, in a democratic society, the relevant health authorities, using sound scientific, medical and epidemiological data, can claim that:

1 a vaccine will protect the great majority of children against an infection which may cause serious disease or be life-threatening, and
2 the risks of serious disease or death following vaccination are *very much less* than those likely to be experienced by some if exposed to the natural infection,

then a child has the right to be vaccinated. The vaccination is beneficial both for the child and for the community. If there are valid medical reasons not to vaccinate, restrictions on travel and exposure to the community by the child may be necessary if there is an outbreak of that disease. Otherwise, it can be argued that the right of the child to be vaccinated should override any opinion to the contrary by the legal guardians of the child.

When we choose to drive or travel in cars, there is no guarantee that we will not suffer a serious or fatal accident at some time. To minimise this risk, we *all* drive on the correct side of the road and we *all* wear seat belts, both for our safety and for the safety of others. The same arguments apply to vaccination.

We understand and appreciate the concerns parents may have about the possible risks of vaccinating young children, and we have tried to address those concerns in this book. But we are very concerned about those in the community who speak and argue strongly against the practice of vaccination. If they are not convinced already by the information presented above and in previous chapters about the efficacy and safety of vaccines, we ask them to consider the following three scenarios.

1   AIDS is now a major disaster especially in developing countries worldwide. Even in Australia, despite the good record of control and the current very expensive multi-drug regimens, deaths still occur from this infection. These drug regimens are not available to the great majority of infected individuals in the world. There is now hope that it should be possible to develop a reasonably effective vaccine.

About half of the world's population are at risk of contracting malaria, and about two million children die each year from this infection. Again there is the prospect of an effective vaccine becoming available.

Chlamydia infections can lead to ectopic pregnancies and pelvic inflammatory disease (PID) in women, a major disease in both developing and developed countries. In the USA, it is the most commonly treated sexually transmitted disease in adolescent females. Efforts to develop an effective vaccine are in progress.

Would members of the anti-vaccination groups argue in principle against the use of vaccines to prevent or greatly ameliorate these infections when effective vaccines become available?

2   There is an annual total of about 300 million cases of hepatitis B virus infections in the world. Though the peak of the incidence of liver cancer resulting from this infection is in middle age, young children can develop cancer from the infection and die. Studies of individuals who acquire HBV infection as infants and young children indicate that 25% will die of either liver cancer or cirrhosis of the liver. The first hepatitis B virus vaccine became available in the early 1980s and is given to babies at birth. The first data (1997) for 6–14-year-old children from a comprehensive trial in Taiwan has shown a 50 per cent reduction in incidence of liver cancer and a 70 per cent reduction in cancer-induced deaths in vaccinated compared to unvaccinated infants, a most encouraging finding.

Each year, 200,000 women are expected to die from cervical cancer. Three phase I clinical trials of candidate vaccines aimed at preventing infection by the causative infectious agents, papilloma viruses, have just concluded with encouraging results.

Would members of the anti-vaccination groups now argue in principle against hepatitis B virus vaccination of babies, or vaccination of pre-adolescent children with a papilloma virus vaccine, when it becomes available?

3   About one in fourteen women in Australia develops breast cancer; the incidence is much higher among women in some families. An Australian immunisation protocol (immuno-therapy) for the treatment of the cancer is undergoing clinical trials. If the preparation proves to be successful in controlling the tumour and even perhaps in inducing regression of the tumour, the next step would be to develop a prophylactic vaccine for administration to pre-adolescent girls.

Sexually transmitted diseases (such as AIDS, pelvic inflammatory disease, and cervical cancer), the major parasitic diseases, especially malaria, and common cancers such as those of the liver, prostate and breast, are the modern global 'pandemics', just as devastating as smallpox and poliomyelitis used to be. Those who are ambivalent about current vaccines may waver because the diseases being prevented are now rare. If they consider that vaccines might in the future prevent the above global diseases, it would help put this technology in perspective, as one of the most important health promoting (disease preventing) measures ever developed.

Postscript

Several items of general interest in the area of vaccinology have arisen in the last few months. The International AIDS Vaccine Initiative (IAVI) was started in New York several years ago by the Rockefeller Foundation with the objective of greatly speeding up the development of vaccines to prevent or control AIDS, as the latter is now generally recognised to cause more deaths worldwide than any other infectious agent or disease. IAVI has steadily grown in international stature and activities, and financial support has come from an increasing number of sources. The major recent development however is that Bill Gates, the CEO of Microsoft and reputedly the richest man in the world, has made a major donation to IAVI in order to speed up HIV vaccine development. Mr Gates has formed the Bill and Melinda Gates Foundation valued (to date, September 1999) in excess of $US17 billion. The foundation has taken on a major role in enhancing the level of vaccination of infants against the common childhood diseases.

At a recent international meeting in Italy chaired by Professor Sir Gustav Nossal (formerly Director of the Walter and Eliza Hall Institute in Melbourne), the focus of the discussion was how to save 40 million young lives over a period of ten years, a project estimated to cost about $US3 billion per year. The aim is to raise the vaccination level of the world's children from its current level of 80 per cent to much closer to 100 per cent by providing not only current but also some oncoming vaccines and, in addition, up-grading the health infrastructure in poor countries. A global coalition—including WHO, UNICEF, major philanthropic foundations, the World Bank and vaccine manufacturers—was formed to achieve this goal, which could rate as 'a major public health achievement of the twenty-first century' (*Science*, 284: 587).

Levels of vaccination with oral polio virus vaccine in several countries are still not high enough to ensure eradication of the virus (see Chapter 7). At the World Health Assembly held in Geneva in May 1999, the countries identified as lagging in this respect pledged their commitment to implementing the necessary increased vaccination activities. Rotary International has offered its 1.4 million volunteers to help in this campaign. It is estimated that an additional $US370 million will be needed to achieve the final goal of eradication, but once this has been achieved, the annual savings in vaccine and immunisation costs will amount to $US1.5 billion. The benefits for millions of as yet unborn children will be very high.

The US Centers for Disease Control and Prevention and the Pan American Health Organization (PAHO) have signed an agreement to work towards the elimination of measles from the western hemisphere (specifically, the Americas) by the year 2000. This follows the publication of PAHO's *Regional Vaccine Initiative* which has been endorsed by all heads of states in the Americas. If measles elimination is achieved on schedule, it will be just nine years since the last case of poliomyelitis caused by native virus was detected in the Americas—a remarkable feat.

In 1998, a report in the *Lancet* (351: 637) suggested there might be an association between immunisation with a measles vaccine (usually MMR) and the later occurrence of inflammatory bowel disease (IBD) and autism. Although an editorial in the same issue of the *Lancet* expressed doubts about the validity of this claim, there was subsequently a small decrease (about 3 per cent) in the uptake of the MMR vaccine in the UK. Such a small dip, however, was still sufficient to allow an epidemic to occur. Since then, five separate epidemiological investigations have found no association between measles vaccination and IBD or autism. In two other studies, measles virus has not been detected in children who had been immunised with MMR and subsequently developed IBD. In two more recent studies (1999), no evidence was found for vaccination with MMR causing autism or IBD (reviewed by Amin, J. and Wong, M. *Communicable Disease Intelligence*. 23: 222). To date, nine separate studies have found no evidence to substantiate the original claim of an association between MMR vaccination and the later occurrence of autism or IBD. This illustrates the care taken to thoroughly investigate a single claim for a causal effect between a vaccination and later adverse effects. Similarly, findings from a 1999 population-based control study (*Nature Medicine*. 5: 964–5) do not support a recently-expressed concern that the Hepatitis B vaccination induces demyelinating diseases, such as multiple sclerosis.

On the other hand, when a new product (following licensure for medical use) is used on very large numbers of recipients for the first time, rare untoward effects *may* become apparent. The new rotavirus vaccine, prepared in the USA, was released for use there in 1998 and has since been administered to 1.5 million children. It was very recently withdrawn from distribution pending further investigation of a side effect called intussesception (a 'telescoping' or restriction of the bowel) detected at the low frequency of about 1 per 10,000 recipients.

Committees of the US Congress are holding hearings on vaccine adverse reactions in general, but the feeling has been expressed that Congressmen are being 'dominated by political concerns and special interests at the expense of sound science' (*Nature Medicine*. 5: 970).

A recent report on the Internet (5 September 1999) described parents in Wales who are deliberately organising 'measles parties' in the belief that exposing children to childhood diseases is the best form of immunisation. A consultant for the local health authority, Dr M. Evans, stated that 'It is one thing to refuse to have your children immunised, but it is quite another to deliberately expose them to harmful diseases'. This example of 'going backwards'—forgetting the hazards of infection with native virus, now seems to be a worldwide problem.

As described in Chapter 11, the practice of vaccination is being applied to prevent or control some non-communicable diseases, such as arthritis, diabetes and some cancers. The application of this approach to other non-communicable diseases is likely to grow, and one (very interesting) possibility is dementia. With the steady ageing of the population in industrial countries, the incidence of the commonest form of dementia, Alzheimer's disease, is increasing and currently, about 20 per cent of the over-80 population in Australia is expected to be affected. The loss of mental capacity of those so affected approaches 100 per cent, and the cost of care becomes a major burden for both society and government. Trying to understand how and why dementia occurs and how to prevent or modify the process is now a very active field of investigation. A general finding is that a protein deposit, called amyloid plaque, builds up in the brains of those affected. In the last few years, mice have been genetically engineered to develop similar plaques in their brains. It has now been shown (*Science.* 285: 175–6) that immunisation of mice with the protein that forms the plaque not only prevents but can even reverse the plaque formation and the consequent damage which occurs to neurones in the brain. It may take a considerable time to see whether such an approach would be effective in preventing or modifying dementia in humans. At least, however, this approach should clarify whether plaque formation is a major contributor to the human disease or simply a by-product of another contributing process. It is another example of the potential of this technology to benefit human welfare.

Appendix 1

Publications on Immunisation (Australia)

The Australian Immunisation Handbook. (7th edition) (1999). National Health and Medical Research Council, Canberra, Commonwealth of Australia. (Available from the Commonwealth Department of Health and Family Services. Tel. 02–6289 1555.

'Understanding childhood immunisation'. Brochure for parents. (Available free from Commonwealth, State and Territory Health Authorities.)

'Immunisation myths and realities'. Brochure for parents and health care professionals. (Available free from Commonwealth, State and Territory Health Authorities.)

Contact telephone numbers for Commonwealth, State and Territory Health Authorities are as follows:

Commonwealth	02 6289 1555
ACT	02 6205 0860
NSW	02 9391 9000
NT	08 8922 8044
Queensland	07 3234 1145
SA	08 8226 6000
Tasmania	03 6233 3762
WA	08 9222 4222

Appendix 2

Revision to the Australian Standard Immunisation Schedule

The Australian Technical Advisory Group on Immunisation (ATAGI) has proposed to introduce a new vaccination schedule that will include provision for the introduction of universal infant hepatitis B vaccination as recommended by the National Health and Medical Research Council (NHMRC). The 'Vaccine' column utilises products which have been registered for supply in Australia as at 11 June 1999 and may be amended from time to time when other products gain registration in Australia. The proposed schedule will become operational following endorsement by the NHMRC at a time to be advised.

The Australian Standard Vaccination Schedule, 2000

Age	Vaccine	
Birth	hepB[a]	
2 months	Path 1[b] DTPa-hepB and Hib and OPV	Path 2[b] DTPa[c] and Hib-hepB and OPV
4 months	DTPa-hepB and Hib OPV	DTPa[c] and Hib-hepB and OPV
6 months	DTPa-hepB and OPV	DTPa[c] and OPV
12 months	MMR and Hib	MMR and Hib-hepB
18 months	DTPa	
4 years	DTPa and MMR and OPV	
10–12 years 1 month later 6 months after 2nd dose	hepB[d] hepB[d] hepB[d]	
15–19 years	Td OPV	
non-immune women who are post-partum and of child bearing age	MMR	
50 years	Td	
50 years and over (Aboriginal and Torres Strait Island people)	Pneumococcal vaccine (every 5 years) Influenza vaccine (every year)	
65 years and over	Pneumococcal vaccine (every 5 years) Influenza vaccine (every year)	

Notes:

a   Hepatitis B vaccine (HBV) should be given to all infants at birth and should not be delayed beyond 7 days after birth. Infants whose mothers are hepatitis B surface antigen positive (HBsAg+ve) should also be given hepatitis B immunoglobulin (HBIG) within 12 hours of birth.

b   When necessary the two paths may be interchanged with regard to their hepatitis B and Hib components. For example, when a child moves interstate, they may change from one path to the other.

c   Wherever possible the same brand of DTPa should be used at 2, 4 and 6 months.

d   Adolescent hepatitis B vaccination is not necessary for those children who have previously received three doses of hepatitis B vaccine.

TRANSITION FROM THE OLD TO THE NEW SCHEDULE

All babies born on or after 1 March 2000 should commence the new schedule. Children born before this date should continue to be vaccinated using the previous schedule. Both the previous schedule and the new schedule are fully interchangeable from 18 months of age.

Disease	Vaccine	Available products
Hepatitis B	hepB	Engerix-B™ or H-B VaxII®
Diphtheria, Tetanus, Pertussis	DTPa	Infanrix™ or Tripacel™
Diphtheria, Tetanus, Pertussis, Hepatitis B	DTPa-hepB	Infanrix-HepB™
Haemophilus influenzae type b	Hib	PedvaxHIB™
Haemophilus influenzae type b Hepatitis B	Hib-hepB	Comvax™
Poliomyelitis	OPV	Polio Sabin™
Measles–Mumps–Rubella	MMR	MMRII® or Priorix™
Diphtheria, Tetanus	Td	ADT Vaccine™
Pneumococcal disease	Pneumococcal vaccine	Pneumovax23®
Influenza	Influenza vaccine	Fluarix™ or Fluvax® or Vaxigrip™ or Flurivin™

Appendix 3

British Immunisation Schedule, 1996

Age	Disease	Vaccine
2 months	Diphtheria-tetanus-whole cell pertussis	DTPw
	Haemophilus influenzae type b vaccine	Hib
	Oral polio vaccine	OPV
3 months	Diphtheria-tetanus-whole cell pertussis	DTPw
	Haemophilus influenzae type b vaccine	Hib
	Oral polio vaccine	OPV
4 months	Diphtheria–tetanus-whole cell pertussis	DTPw
	Haemophilus influenzae type b vaccine	Hib
	Oral polio vaccine	OPV
12–15 months	Measles-mumps-rubella vaccine	MMR
3–5 years	Diphtheria-tetanus	DT
	Measles-mumps-rubella vaccine	MMR
	Oral polio vaccine	OPV
13–18 years	Diphtheria-tetanus	DT
	Oral polio vaccine	OPV

Appendix 4

Standard US Immunisation Schedule, August 1999

Age	Disease	Vaccine
0–2 months 1–4 months 6–18 months	Hepatitis B	hep b
2 months 4 months 6 months 15–18 months 4–6 years	Diphtheria-tetanus-acellular-pertussis	DTPa
2 months 4 months 6 months 12–15 months	*Haemophilus influenzae* type b	Hib
2 months 4 months 6–18 months 4–6 years	Polio	Injectable polio vaccine (IPV)
12–15 months 4–6 years	Measles-mumps-rubella	MMR
12–18 months (for susceptible persons over 13 years, 2 doses one month apart)	Varicella	varicella

Glossary

adjuvant A preparation which may be added to a vaccine to improve the immune response to the vaccine. Alum is still the only adjuvant licensed for general use. They are mainly used with subunit and conjugate vaccines.

adverse effects of vaccination These are discussed in Chapter 6.

affinity maturation Refers to the fact that antibody produced later following immunisation/vaccination has a higher affinity (binds more strongly to the antigen) compared to antibody produced early during the immune response. The antibody-secreting cells (B lymphocytes) or circulating B memory lymphocytes compete for antigen (bound to the surface of follicular dendritic cells in germinal centres). Those producing antibody or with antibody receptors of higher affinity compete more effectively and go on to mature further. Unsuccessful cells die and are phagocytosed (eaten).

alleles/polymorphism Alternative DNA sequences of the same gene which change the structure of part of the protein product slightly, but conserve the basic function of the whole molecule are called alleles. A population of individuals expressing different alleles of the same gene is said to be polymorphic for that gene. The term is used mainly for the major histocompatibility complex (MHC) protein antigens.

amino acids These are the basic chemical building blocks of proteins.

antibiotics Compounds which prevent the growth of bacteria and are widely used to cure infections.

antibody An antibody (immunoglobulin) is a protein produced by B lymphocytes in response to immunisation/vaccination with a foreign substance or antigen (part of a virus, bacterium or parasite). The antibody binds to the antigen and in so doing may neutralise the infectivity of the infectious agent. The antigen:antibody complex is phagocytosed (eaten) by cells such as macrophages and so destroyed. The simplest types of antibodies are IgG, IgA, and IgE (Ig for immunoglobulin) and are composed of two light (L) and two heavy (H) peptide chains. L and H chains have constant and very variable regions (sequences).

antigen-binding site of antibodies The intricate three-dimensional folding of the variable regions of an H and L chain at one end of the LH segment of an antibody which bind to part of the surface of an antigen. The part of the antigen so complexing with the antibody is called an epitope. The epitope can be a continuous sequence of amino acids (a peptide) or of sugars (carbohydrate) or a discontinuous sequence formed by adjacent chains of peptides or carbohydrates. The antigen-binding site 'sees' a two-dimensional shape.

The epitope 'seen' by the T lymphocyte receptor is also a two-dimensional shape, but in this case, it is a peptide (from an antigen) held in the groove at the end of the major histocompatibility complex (MHC) antigen molecule. Thus, part of the end of the MHC molecule *and* the embedded peptide form the epitope.

antigen/self antigen/immunogen An antigen is an organic molecule which can be recognised by the immune system, either as being part of the body (self) or foreign. It is usually a sequence of amino acids—a short sequence is called a peptide, and a longer sequence is called a protein. It may also be a sequence of sugar (carbohydrate) molecules. A short sequence is called an oligosaccharide and a long sequence is called a polysaccharide. It may be a combination of a protein and oligosaccharides, called a glycoprotein. If it induces an immune response following administration to a live host, it is called an *immunogen* (potentially capable of inducing immunity). From the point of view of making vaccines, many antigens of interest are constituents of viruses, bacteria or parasites.

During foetal life, we become tolerant to our own antigens and generally do not make an immune response to them (Chapter 4). If we do, this is called autoimmunity (immunity to self, Chapter 10).

apoptosis The term used to describe a process of biologically planned cell death. This is completely normal and contrasts with the cell death which occurs due to injury (burns, trauma, etc.), called necrosis. In a middle-aged person, most of the cells in the body would be only a few years old, as most cells 'wear out' and need to be replaced relatively often. Much of the energy we expend in life is to get rid of old cells and make new ones.

attenuation The process of modifying a virus or bacterium so as to reduce its virulence (disease-inducing ability), while retaining its ability to induce a strong immune response (immunogenicity).

autoimmunity An immune reaction against the body's own components.

B lymphocyte (or cell) Bone marrow-derived, 'white' blood cells which travel to and from the lymphoid tissues via lymph vessels (hence the name). The cells have an antibody (immunoglobulin, Ig) receptor on their surface. When this reacts specifically with an antigen, the B cell is 'activated' and will differentiate to become an antibody-secreting cell (ASC), producing anti bodies only of that particular specificity. The common Igs are IgM, IgG, IgE, and IgA. Two molecules of IgA, linked together, can be secreted from a mucosal surface as a dimer, secretory or s.IgA. IgG, IgE and IgA have two antigen-binding sites whereas IgM has ten such sites.

Base Refers to the bases adenine (A), thymine (T), guanine (G) and cytosine (C) in DNA. T is replaced by uracil (U) in RNA.

BCG Bacille Calmette Guerin, the attenuated tuberculosis vaccine.

CD Cluster of differentiation, refers to markers on the surface of cells, such as CD4 and CD8 on lymphocytes.

cDNA A complementary (copy) DNA sequence. This is the DNA sequence obtained by copying the sequence of bases in an RNA by a 'reverse transcriptase' enzyme.

chemokines Small polypeptides that are produced by cells like macrophages. They attract phagocytic cells, causing their migration to sites of infection.

chromosome A long, double-stranded DNA molecule, which is circular in bacteria. In higher cells, it is linear and complexed with proteins called 'histones', forming a complex called chromatin.

clinical trials After a potential vaccine has been shown to be safe and effective in experimental animals, it is tested in human volunteers. Phase I trials are carried out on a small number primarily to test for safety; phase II on a larger number to check for safety and immunogenicity and phase III trials, sometimes on very large numbers, to check that it protects against disease (efficacy).

clonal selection As B lymphocytes formed in the bone marrow mature, they express antibody (immunoglobulin or Ig) molecules at their surface, called an Ig receptor (usually IgM). A single cell expresses only Igs of a *single antigen-binding specificity*. A foreign antigen entering the body binds only to cells expressing closely fitting (complementary) receptors—a Darwinian type selection. These cells become activated, divide and differentiate to become antibody-secreting cells (ASCs). To do this and secrete other classes of antibody (e.g. IgG), they interact with activated T cells. If this doesn't happen, only IgM is secreted. After activation, some cells become memory cells and they express other Igs, (IgG, IgA or IgE). During differentiation which takes place in lymphoid follicles/germinal centres, extensive mutation of sequences in the antigen-binding sites can occur. This can result in *affinity maturation* of the Ig receptors and of the secreted antibody. Cells with receptors which best fit the antigen are selected to survive and make antibody of high affinity to the antigen. Others die by apoptosis.

constant/variable regions of antibodies The polypeptide light (L) and heavy (H) chains of antibodies have regions where the amino acid sequence is largely constant, and regions where there is great variation in the sequence. The variable regions of both chains interact and form the antigen-binding site. Different parts of the L and H chains, acting together, contain sequences which allow the antibody molecule, usually complexed with antigen, to bind to different cells such as macrophages.

CTLs See **cytotoxic T lymphocytes**

cytokines/interleukins/interferons Protein molecules secreted by different cells which, when they combine with a specific receptor on other cells, can influence the behaviour of that cell, such as activation, replication or differentiation. Cytokine is the general name used for these proteins. Interleukins refer to cytokines influencing the behaviour of lymphocytes. Interferon is one kind of cytokine. T lymphocytes in particular make and secrete a wide variety of cytokines. Cytokines, unlike hormones which can act on distant targets in the body, act over very short distances.

cytoplasm. That part of the cell outside the nucleus and containing other structures such as mitochondria.

cytotoxic T lymphocytes (CTLs) Sometimes called 'killer' T lymphocytes. They possess the plasma membrane marker, CD8. The T cell receptor (TCR) recognises a complex of peptide and class I MHC molecule on the surface of an antigen-presenting cell (APC). This activates the cell and once mature, it will kill any cell expressing that complex. Usually, such 'target cells' are infected with a virus, bacterium or parasite, the peptide coming from the breakdown of a newly synthesised foreign protein.

dendritic cells These cells have long 'branches' called dendrites, which gives them a large surface area. Those near the skin are called Langerhans cells and take foreign antigen from the periphery to the 'draining' lymphoid tissues where they present the antigen to T lymphocytes, and hence are called antigen-presenting cells (APCs). They 'process' the antigen, breaking it down to peptides, some of which combine with major histocompatibility antigen. The complex is recognised by the T cell receptor (TCR). They also produce co-stimulator molecules which are necessary for T cell activation.

DNA Deoxyribonucleic acid is the molecule which carries genetic information. embodied in the sequence of the bases adenine (A), thymine (T), cytosine (C) and guanine (G), which are linked together by phosphodiester bonds. In its native form, it is a very long, base-paired polymer, two strands of which intertwine to form a double helix consisting of millions of bases. A pairs with T and G with C. A single human chromosome contains many millions of bases.

domain The term is used to describe a structural or functional part of a protein. For example, the constant region of the IgG antibody consists of three domains. The variable region is one domain.

endemic A region where an infectious disease is always present

enzyme A protein which catalyses (greatly speeds up) a biochemical reaction.

epidemics Occur when the level of non-immune, ('susceptible') people in a community increases to the extent that transmission of an infectious agent occurs more readily and there is a surge of new infections in the susceptible group. Epidemics may occur frequently with highly infectious agents like measles (see Figure 5.2), but not at all where transmission of the infection between people is very low, e.g., tetanus. See also **pandemics** and **herd immunity**.

FDA Federal Drug Administration, USA.

FDC Follicular dendritic cells (meaning cells with many long 'arms' and hence a very large surface area) present in the follicles of lymphoid tissues. Unlike dendritic cells which are very mobile, FDCs are only present in the follicles of lymphoid tissue. Antigen, as antigen/antibody complexes, binds to the surface of FDCs and may persist there for very long periods. Differentiating B lymphocytes with the best binding receptors are selected by the bound antigen to become antibody-secreting cells (ASCs). Memory B lymphocytes may also react with the FDC-bound antigen and become ASCs. The nett result is the continuing production of antibody specific for that antigen. While this very active process is ongoing, the follicles are termed germinal centres (GC). The GC can thus be envisioned as the site where the fittest, differentiating B lymphocytes with the highest affinity receptors for the antigen survive and become ASCs. Those cells not selected by antigen in this way die by apoptosis.

gametes Cells of the reproductive system, spermatozoa and ova (eggs).

genetic engineering The ability to transfer DNA coding for important antigens into other cells which can then produce the protein vaccine, or into other attenuated live agent vaccines, which can then be used to induce an immune response to the antigen encoded by the transferred DNA. DNA coding for specific antigens is now being assessed as a vaccine (Chapter 9).

genome Refers to the complete set of genes in a cell or infectious agent.

germinal centre See **FDC**.

H chain The heavy (larger) polypeptide chain of an antibody molecule.

haptens Chemically synthesised molecules which are large enough (e.g., derivatives of benzine) to be recognised by antibodies. They are not immunogenic per se (cannot by themselves induce antibody formation). If conjugated (attached to) a foreign protein, the complex is immunogenic, the antibodies so formed recognising hapten and the protein 'carrier'. This principle is used in the composition of conjugate vaccines. It allows babies to respond much better to the vaccine and hence to deal with pathogenic bacteria.

helper T lymphocytes T lymphocytes which 'help' B lymphocytes make antibodies. They are characterised by the cell membrane 'marker' CD4. When activated following interaction with an antigen-presenting cell (APC) expressing peptide/class II MHC antigen complexes, the T cell secretes different cytokines which 'help' the replication and differentiation of B lymphocytes and also sometimes help in the differentiation of CD8+ T lymphocytes to become CTLs.

herd immunity Occurs when the proportion of people immune to an infection is sufficiently high that transmission of the infection to susceptibles is low. For a highly infectious virus like measles, over 95 per cent of people need to be immune in order for a population to have herd immunity; for smallpox, the figure was about 80 per cent. The task of eradicating smallpox was therefore less demanding than is required to eradicate measles.

HLA Human leucocyte antigen, the name given to MHC antigens in humans.

hybridoma A normal B lymphocyte can be 'immortalised' by the technique of fusing it with a continuously dividing B tumour lymphocyte, to create a cell—a hybridoma—which continuously secretes antibody of the desired specificity. Large quantities of specific antibodies can be made in this way. It was one of the last pieces of evidence proving the Clonal Selection Theory proposed by Burnet.

Ig Abbreviation for immunoglobulin.

IgM, IgG, IgE, IgA, IgD The different classes of immunoglobulins distinguished by size (number of H and L chains) and by sequence differences in their H chain constant regions which allow them to have different functions such as attaching to the plasma membranes of different cells.

immunisation The process of administering a foreign substance in order to induce an immune response. For example, the antibody so produced may be needed for an experimental purpose in a laboratory. Both immunisation and vaccination are used to describe the process of inducing an immune response in order to protect a host against an infectious organism.

immunocompetent A lymphocyte is said to be immunocompetent when it has the ability to recognise and respond to an antigen.

immunoglobulin Formal term for an antibody molecule, often abbreviated to Ig.

interferons (IFNs) These are naturally occurring proteins with anti-viral and immunoregulatory activities. There are two classes of interferons; alpha (IFNα) and beta (IFNβ) are similar molecules whereas gamma interferon (IFNγ) is quite different and is sometimes known as immune IFN as it is also produced by some activated T lymphocyes. Their major role is to inhibit viral replication.

killer T cell Sometimes used as a less formal term than cytotoxic T lymphocyte (CTL).

L chain Light (smaller) peptide chain of an antibody molecule.

lymphoid organs The bone marrow and the thymus are regarded as primary lymphoid organs because that is where the lymphocytes develop and become immunocompetent. The spleen and different lymph nodes are called secondary lymphoid organs because that is where lymphocytes meet with antigen and become effector cells.

MHC Major histocompatibility complex antigen is essentially a self marker on most cells of the body. There are two classes, I and II. Class I MHC molecules associate with peptides from foreign antigens such as viruses; class II MHC molecules associate with peptides from non-infectious antigens, including self proteins. MHC molecules are the most polydisperse (ubiquitous) group of molecules in the body, and they have a crucial role in the immune response which is described in Chapters 4 and 5.

mRNA Messenger RNA is the mechanism whereby information coded in the DNA of a cell is transcribed into the RNA which in turn is translated into protein.

mutation Change in a DNA base sequence so that when the DNA is replicated, the mutation in the base sequence is copied into the progeny DNA molecules.

natural killer (NK) cells Part of the innate system. Major producers of the interferons, which are active in controlling viral replication until the adaptive system comes into play. They can also kill tumour cells if the level of class I MHC antigen on these cells is down-regulated

nucleic acids The chemical term for DNA and RNA.

nucleotides The basic chemical building blocks of nucleic acids. See **bases**.

nucleus The membrane-bounded organelle within a higher cell which contains the complete set of chromosomes. This would usually be a diploid (double) number for somatic (body) cells, but half that (haploid number) for a male or female gamete (sperm or egg).

opsonisation A complex of antigen with antibody which is more readily phagocytosed (eaten) by macrophages than the free antigen.

organelle A complex structure within the cytoplasm of a higher cell and which has a specialised function.

pandemic A worldwide epidemic of an infectious agent, e.g., HIV/AIDS or influenza.

plasmid A circular double-stranded molecule of DNA which replicated independently of the chromsomal DNA in bacteria. Chimeric plasmids containing DNA sequences coding for different foreign antigens are used as candidate vaccines.

peptide A 'string' of amino acids linked together by covalent (special) bonds. A long peptide chain is called a protein.

When a protein is degraded by a proteolytic enzyme (protease), it is usually said to be broken down into peptides.

phagocyte/phagocytosis Phagocytes are white blood cells which can engulf or eat (phagocytose) and digest particles such as bacteria or other cellular debris (such as cells which have died by apoptosis). Coating bacteria or viruses with specific antibody (opsonisation) enhances their phagocytosis. Macrophages are major phagocytes in the body.

point mutation Refers to a single base change in the nucleic acid.

protein A long polymer of amino acids joined by peptide (covalent) bonds, usually 100–300 amino acid residues in length.

reverse transcriptase An enzyme which copies an RNA base sequence into a DNA base sequence. It is present in retroviruses such as HIV.

reverse transcription The synthesis of a complementary copy of DNA (termed cDNA) from a single-stranded RNA template by a reverse transcriptase.

RNA Ribonucleic acids are usually single-stranded complementary copies of selected stretches of DNA sequences. They contain four nucleotide bases, adenine (A), uracil (U), cytosine (C) and guanine (G). In RNA, U is functionally equivalent to A in DNA. Viruses contain either RNA or DNA as their genetic material.

somatic cell All cells in the body except those involved in reproduction (sperm and eggs) which are called gametes. See also **nucleus.**

somatic hypermutation When B lympocytes are activated and differentiate, extensive mutation can occur in the variable region of the genes coding for immunoglobulins. The rate of mutation can be up to a million times faster than background levels. The process occurs almost exclusively in the germinal centres of lymphoid tissues. In this way, those cells making antibody of higher affinity are chosen by localised antigen to become antibody secreting cells (plasma cells).

STDs Sexually transmitted diseases.

T lymphocyte Precursor T cells migrate from the bone marrow to the thymus gland (T for thymus) where they mature and many cells with specificity to host antigens are eliminated. The mature T cells are mobile, circulating in lymphoid tissues via lymph vessels, and in the blood. The T cell receptors (TCR) for recognising antigen are rather similar to immunoglobulins, but instead of recognising intact antigen, they recognise degradation products (peptides) bound to MHC antigens at a cell surface. There are two major types. T cells with the surface marker, CD4, help B cells make antibody (are called helper cells) and secrete a distinct pattern of cytokines. T cells with the surface marker, CD8, have the ability to kill infected cells and are called cytotoxic T lymphocytes (CTLs) or simple killer T cells, and secrete a different pattern of cytokines.

trachoma Blindness due to repeated chlamydia infection of the eye.

vaccination The term most widely used to describe the process of immunisation for the special purpose of protecting against disease caused by an infectious agent. The term is derived from vaccinia (cowpox virus, from *vacca*, a cow), the virus used by Jenner to protect against a subsequent smallpox infection. The term is now widely used to describe immunisation to protect against any infection.

vaccines There are three main types: live, attenuated agents; inactivated whole agents; and subunit preparations (only part of the agent), including toxoids, and conjugate vaccines. Current vaccines are described in Chapter 3. Newer approaches to vaccine development are described in Chapter 9.

WHO The World Health Organization, with headquarters in Geneva.

viraemia The presence in the blood of free virus, i.e., non-cell associated, after an infection has occurred.

References and further reading

CHAPTER 1 INFECTIOUS DISEASES OF HUMANS

Burnet, M. and White, D.O. (1972). *Natural History of Infectious Disease*. Cambridge University Press, Cambridge.

Coker, R. (1998). Lessons from New York's tuberculosis epidemic. *Br. Med. J.* 317: 616.

Diamond, J. (1997), *Guns, Germs and Steel*. Jonathan Cape, London.

Fenner, F. (1998). Sociocultural changes and infectious disease. In: *Infectious Disease in Humans*. Howard Florey Centenary Symposium. ed. B. Furnass, Aussie Print: 21–31.

Gerbase, A.C., Rowley, J.T. and Mertens, T.E. (1988). Global epidemiology of sexually transmitted diseases. *Lancet* 351; suppl. 2–4.

Merlino, J. (1998). Detecting enterococci and vancomycin resistance. *Today's Life Science*. 10 (9): 37–39.

Mims, C. (1998). Modes of transmission of infectious agents. In: *Infectious Disease in Humans*. Howard Florey Centenary Symposium. ed. B. Furnass, Aussie Print: 32–40.

Oldstone, M.A.B. (1998). *Viruses, Plagues and History*. Oxford University Press, New York.

Preston, R. (1998). Annals of warfare. The bioweaponeers. *The New Yorker*. March 9.

Spratt, B.G. (ed.) (1988). Resurgent/emerging infectious diseases. *British Medical Bulletin*. 54 (3): 523–765.

World Health Organization (1988). Animals and human health. *World Health*, Geneva, 51(4): 1–31.

World Health Report (1998). World Health Organization, Geneva.

Zinsser, H. (1935). *Rats, Lice and History*. Blue Ribbon Books and Little, Brown and Co, Boston.

CHAPTER 2 A SHORT HISTORY OF VACCINES AND VACCINATION

Baxby, D. (1999). The end of smallpox. *History Today.* 49: 14–16.

Fenner, F., Henderson, D.A., Arita, I., Jezek, Z. and Ladnyi, I.D. (1988). *Smallpox and its Eradication.* World Health Organization, Geneva.

Hopkins, D.R. (1983). *Princes and Peasants. Smallpox in History.* University of Chicago Press, Chicago.

Parish, H.J. (1965). *A History of Immunization.* Livingston Ltd, Edinburgh.

Plotkin, S.L. and Plotkin, S.A. (1999). A short history of vaccination. In: *Vaccines.* eds S.A. Plotkin and W.A. Orenstein. W.B. Saunders Co., Philadelphia.

Wilson, G. S. (1967). *The Hazards of Immunization.* Athlone Press, London.

CHAPTER 3 CURRENT VACCINES AND VACCINATION PROCEDURES

The Australian Immunisation Handbook (1999). 7th edition, NHMRC, Canberra.

Australian Society for Geriatric Medicine. Position statement No. 7. Immunisation of Older People

Children's Vaccine Initiative Forum. CVI Secretariat, World Health Organization, Geneva, Published thrice yearly.

Henderson, R.H. 1994. Vaccination: successes and challenges. In: *Vaccination and World Health.* eds F.T. Cutts and P.G. Smith. Wiley, Chichester: 3–16.

National Institutes of Health (1998). *The Jordan Report: Accelerated Development of Vaccines.* NIAID, Washington.

Siegrist, C.A., Dodet, B. and Lambert, P.H. (1999). Immunity in early life, an introduction. (A series of papers from a meeting held in November 1998). *Vaccine,* 16, nos 14/15.

Spratt, B.G. (ed.). (1988) Resurgent/emerging infectious diseases. *British Medical Bulletin.* 54(3): 523–765.

World Health. Magazine of the World Health Organization, published monthly. (Ceased publication in 1999).

CHAPTER 4 HOW VACCINES WORK: THE IMMUNE RESPONSE TO INFECTIOUS AGENTS AND VACCINES

Ada, Gordon L. and Nossal, Sir Gustav (1987). The clonal-selection theory. *Scientific American.* 255: 62–69.

Ada, G. and Ramsay, A. (1997). *Vaccines, Vaccination and the Immune Response.* Lippincott-Raven, Philadelphia. 1–247.

Burnet, F.M. (1957). A modification of Jerne's theory of antibody production using the concept of clonal selection. *Aust. J. Science.* 20: 67–69. (This paper is a great example of concise scientific writing).

Haraguchi, S., et al. (1998). Interleukin 12 deficiency associated with recurrent infections. *Proc. Natl. Acad. Sci. USA.* 95: 13125–9.

Janeway, C.A. and Travers, P. (1997). *Immunobiology. The Immune System in Health and Disease.* Current Biology Ltd/Garland Publishing Inc., New York and London.

Paul, W.E. (1991). *Immunology. Recognition and Response.* Readings from *Scientific American.* 1–168.

CHAPTER 5 VACCINE EFFICACY AND THE VARIATION IN INDIVIDUAL RESPONSES

Cutts, F.T., and Smith, P.G., (eds) (1994). *Vaccination and World Health.* John Wiley and Sons, Chichester.

Gerbase, A.C. et al. (1998). Global epidemiology of sexually transmitted diseases. *Lancet.* 351 (supplement III): 2–4.

Glass, R.I., Gentsel, J. and Smith, J.C. (1994). Rotavirus vaccines: success by reassortment? *Science.* 265: 1389–91.

McNicholl, J.M. and Cuenco, K.T. (1999). Host genes and infectious disease. HIV, other pathogens and a public health perspective. *Am. J. of Prev. Med. 16: 141–54.*

Moxon, E.R. (1998) Applications of molecular microbiology to vaccinology. *Lancet.* 350: 1240–44.

National Institutes of Health (1998). *The Jordan Report: Accelerated Development of Vaccines.* NIAID, Washington.

Raoult, D. (1998). Return of the plagues. *Lancet.* 352; suppl. IV: 18.

CHAPTER 6 VACCINE SAFETY

Barraff, J.K., Shields, W.D., et al. (1998). Infants and children with convulsions and hypotonic/hyporesponsive episodes following DTP immunisation; follow-up evaluation. *Pediatrics.* 81: 801–5.

Braun, M.M. and Ellenbergy, S.S. (1997). Descriptive epidemiology of adverse events after immunization: Reports to the Vaccine Adverse Event Reporting System (VAERS), 1991–1994. *Journal of Pediatrics.* 131(4): 529–535.

Chen, R.T. and 14 others plus the Vaccines Safety Datalink Team (1997). Vaccine safety datalink project: A new tool for improving safety monitoring in the United States. *Pediatrics.* 99(6): 765–773.

Chen, R.T., Rastogi, S.C., Mullen, J.R., et al. (1994). The vaccine adverse reporting systems (VAERS). *Vaccine.* 12(6): 542–550.

Gangarosa, E.J., Galaska, M.A., Wolfe, C.R., et al. (1998). Impact of antivaccine movements on pertussis control: the untold story. *Lancet.* 35: 356—61.

Greco, D., Salmaso, S., Mastrantonio, P., et al. (1996). A controlled trial of two acellular vaccines and one whole-cell vaccine against pertussis. *N. Engl. J. Med.* 334: 341–48.

Griffin, M.R., Ray, W.A., Livengood, J.R., Schafnem, W. (1988). Risk of sudden infant death syndrome after immunisation with diphtheria-tetanus-pertussis vaccine. *N. Engl. J. Med.* 319: 618—23.

Gustafsson, L., Hallande, H.O., Olin, P. et al. (1996). A controlled trial of a two-component acellular, a five-component acellular, and a whole-cell pertussis vaccine. *N. Engl. J. Med.* 334: 349–55.

Howson, C.P., Howe, C.J., Fineberg, H.V., (eds) (1994). Adverse effects of pertussis and rubella vaccines—a report of the committee to review the adverse consequences of pertussis and rubella vaccines. Institute of Medicine, National Academy Press, Washington DC.

Kemp, T., Pearce, N., Fitzharris, P., Craine, J., et al. (1997). Is infant immunisation a risk factor for childhood asthma or allergy? *Epidemiology.* 8: 678—80.

Leask, J-A. and Chapman, S. (1998). 'An attempt to swindle nature': press anti-immunisation reportage 1993–1997. *ANZJ. Pub. Health.* 22: 17–26.

Miller, D., Madge, N., Diamond, J., et al. (1993). Pertussis immunisation and serious acute neurological illnesses in children. *Br. Med. J.* 307: 1171–5.

Nolan, T., Hogg, G., Darcy, M-A., et al. (1997). Primary course immunogenicity and reactogenicity of a new diphtheria-tetanus-whole cell pertussis vaccine (DTPw). *J. Paediatr. Child Health.* 33: 413–17.

Peltola, H. and Heinonen, O.P. (1986). Frequency of true adverse reactions to measles-mumps-rubella vaccine. A double-blind placebo-controlled trial in twins. *Lancet.* 1: 939–42.

Peltola, H., Patja, A., Leinikki, P., et al. (1998). No evidence for measles, mumps and rubella vaccine-associated inflammatory bowel disease or autism in a 14 year prospective study. *Lancet.* 351: 1327–8.

Ramsay, M.E., Miller, E., Ashworth, L.A.E. (1995). Adverse events and antibody response to accelerated immunisation in term and preterm infants. *Arch. Dis. Child.* 72: 230–2.

Stratton, K.R., Howe, C.J., Johnston, R.B. (eds) (1994). *Adverse Events Associated with Childhood Vaccines: Evidence Bearing on Causality.* National Academy Press, Washington.

Wakefield, A.J., Murch, S.H., Anthony, A., et al. (1998). Ileal-lymphoidnodular hyperplasia, non-specific colitis and pervasive development disorder in children. *Lancet.* 351: 637–41.

World Health Organization. Special program for vaccines and immunization (1998). Guidelines for implementing a surveillance system for adverse events following immunization (AEFI). Geneva, WHO.

CHAPTER 7 THE CROWNING ACHIEVEMENT—THE ERADICATION/ELIMINATION OF SOME HUMAN INFECTIOUS DISEASES

Dowdle, W.R. and Hopkins, D.R. (1998). *The Eradication of Infectious Diseases.* John Wiley and Sons, Chichester: 1–218.

Fenner, F. (1984). Smallpox, 'The most deadful scourge of the human species.' Its global spread and recent eradication. *Med. J. Aust.* 141: 841–6.

Fenner, F., Henderson, D.A., Arita, I., Jezek, Z., Ladnyi, I.D. (1988). Smallpox and its eradication. World Health Organization, Geneva. 1–1460.

Plotkin, S.A., Katz, M., Cordero, J.F. (1999). The eradication of rubella. *J. American Medical Assoc.* 281: 561–2.

World Health Organization. (1998). Global disease elimination and eradication as public health strategies. *Bulletin of the World Health Organization*, Supplement no. 2 to Volume 76.

World Health Organization, Weekly Epidemiological Reports. These fairly regularly have reports updating progress in the above campaigns. Example, 22 January, 1999.

CHAPTER 8 ADDRESSING PARENTAL CONCERNS

Bond, L., Nolan, T., Pattison, P., Carlin, J. (1998). Vaccine preventable diseases and immunisations: a qualitative study of mothers' perceptions of severity, susceptibility, benefits and barriers. *ANZJ Pub. Health.* 22: 441–6.

Bond, L. (1999). 'The influence of consumers' perceptions of risk, targeted interventions and the effectiveness of incentives on child immunisation uptake'. PhD thesis. University of Melbourne.

Commonwealth Department of Health and Family Services (1988). *Immunisation Myths and Realities.* CAHFS, Canberra. (The statement 'The Medical Association for Homeopathy recommends orthodox immunisation with standard vaccines' can be found on page 17.)

Frisch, D. and Baron, J. (1998). Ambiguity and rationality. *J. Behavioural Decision Making.* 1: 149–57.

Iversky, A. and Kahneman, D. (1981). The framing of decisions and the psychology of choice. *Science.* 211:453–8.

World Health Organization (1999). Pertussis vaccines. *World Epidemiological Record.* 74: 137–43.

CHAPTER 9 NEW APPROACHES TO VACCINE DEVELOPMENT AND IMMUNISATION PRACTICES

General

Arakawa, T. and Langridge, W.H.R. (1998). Plants are not just passive creatures. *Nature Med. 4: 550–1.*

Enserink, M. (1999). Gene may promise new route to potent vaccines. *Science.* 284: 883.

Husband, A.J., et al. (eds) (1997). *Mucosal Solutions. Advances in Mucosal Immunology.* Volumes 1 and 2. University of Sydney.

Mason, H.S., et al. (1998). Subunit vaccines produced and delivered in transgenic plants as 'edible vaccines'. *Research in Immunology,* Institut Pasteur/Elsevier. 149: 71–4.

Specific

Hanke, T., et al. (1998). Enhancement of MHC class I-restricted peptide-specific T cell induction by a DNA prime/MVA boost vaccination regimen. *Vaccine.* 16: 439–45.

Horner, A.A., et al. (1998). Immunostimulatory DNA is a potent mucosal adjuvant. *Cell. Immunology.* 190: 77–82.

Kent, S.J., et al. (1998). Enhanced T-cell immunogenicity and protective efficacy of a human immunodeficiency virus type 1 vaccine regimen consisting of consecutive priming with DNA and boosting with recombinant fowlpox virus. *J. Vir.* 72: 10180–8.

Leong, K.H., et al. (1995). Generation of enhanced immune responses by consecutive immunisation with DNA and recombinant fowlpox viruses. In: *Vaccines, '95.* eds F. Brown, R. Chanock, E. Norrby. Cold Spring Harbor, Laboratory Press, New York: 327–31.

Mason, H.S., et al. (1996). Expression of Norwalk virus capsid protein in transgenic tobacco and potato and its oral immunogenicity in mice. *Proc. Natl. Acad. Sci.* 93: 5335–40.

Modelska, A., et al. (1998). Immunization against rabies with plant-derived antigen. *Proc. Natl. Acad. Sci.* 95: 2481–5.

Pisetsky, D. S. (1996). Immune activation by bacterial DNA: a new genetic code. *Immunity.* 5: 303–10.

Robinson, H.L. and 16 others. (1999). Neutralising antibody-independent containment of immunodeficiency virus challenges by DNA priming and recombinant pox virus booster immunizations. *Nature Med.* 5: 526–34.

Schneider, J., et al. (1998). Enhanced immunogenicity for CD8+ T cell induction and complete protective efficacy of malaria DNA vaccination by boosting with modified vaccinia virus Ankara. *Nature Med.* 4: 397–402.

Plants

Hammond J., McGarvey, P., Yusikov, Y. (eds) (1999). Plant biotechnology. New products and applications. *Contemporary Topics in Microbiology and Immunology.* 240: 1–196.

Ma, J.K-C., et al. (1998). Characterization of a recombinant plant monoclonal secretory antibody and preventive immunotherapy in humans. *Nature Med.* 4: 601–6.

Tacket, C.O., et al. (1998). Immunogenicity in humans of a recombinant bacterial antigen delivered in a transgenic potato. *Nature Med. 4: 6079.*

CHAPTER 10 THE CHALLENGE OF MAKING VACCINES AGAINST HIV, MALARIA AND CHLAMYDIA

General

Chlamydia genome map complete. Implications for vaccine development. (1998/9). *Health Horizons.* 36: 12.

Campbell, L.A., Kuo, C-C, Grayston, J.T. (1998). *Chlamydia pneumoniae* and cardiovascular disease. *Emerging Infectious Diseases.* 4: 571–9.

Cohen, J. (1999). AIDS virus traced to chimps. *Science.* 283: 772–3.

Various authors. (1998). *World Health.* World Health Organization, Geneva. United against malaria, May–June, 1–31; Animals and health, July–August, 1–31.

World Health Organization, Weekly Epidemiological Report, 1999. 74: 105–12.

Taylor, H. (1999). Towards the global elimination of trachoma. *Nature Med.* 5: 492–3.

Specific

Ada, G.L. (1988). Prospects for HIV vaccines. *J. AIDS.* 1: 295–303.

Ada, G.L. and McElrath, M.J. (1996). Perspective. HIV type–1 vaccine-induced cytotoxic T cell responses: potential role in vaccine efficacy. *AIDS Res. Hum. Retroviruses.* 13: 243–8.

Ada, G.L. (1999). Challenges of chronic persisting infections of global importance for vaccine developers. In *Biosciences, 2000.* ed. C.A. Pasternak, Imperial College Press, London: 93–108

Bernard, N.F. and 3 others. (1999). Human immunodeficieincy virus (HIV)-specific cytotoxic T lymphocyte activity in HIV-exposed seronegative persons. *J. Infect. Dis.* 179: 538–47.

Goh, W.C. and 10 others. (1999). Protection against human immunodeficiency virus type 1 infection in persons with repeated exposure: evidence for T cell immunity in the absence of inherited CCR5 coreceptor defects. *J. Infect. Dis.* 179: 548–57.

Kent, S.J., et al. (1998). Enhanced T-cell immunogenicity and protective efficacy of a human immunodeficiency virus type 1 vaccine regimen consisting of consecutive priming with DNA and boosting with recombinant fowlpox virus. *J. Virol.* 72: 10180–8.

Letvin, N.L. (1998). Progress in the development of an HIV vaccine. *Science.* 280: 1875–80.

Montefiori, D.C. and Moore, J. P. (1999). Magic of the Occult? *Science.* 283: 336–7 (and associated references).

Robinson H.L. and 16 others. (1999). Neutralising antibody-independent containment of immunodeficiency virus challenges by DNA priming and recombinant pox virus booster immunizations. *Nature Med.* 5: 526–34.

Schmitz, J.E., et al. (1999). Control of viremia in simian immunodeficiency virus infection by CD8+ lymphocytes. *Science.* 283: 857–60.

Schneider, J., et al. (1998). Enhanced immunogenicity for CD8+T cell induction and complete protective efficacy of malaria DNA vaccination by boosting with modified vaccinia virus Ankara. *Nature Med.* 4: 397–402.

Su, H., Messer, R., Whitmire, W., et al. (1998). Vaccination against Chlamydial genital tract infection after immunization with dendritic cells pulsed ex vivo with non-viable *Chlamydiae. J. Exp. Med.* 188: 809–18.

Weiss, R.A. and Wranghams, R.W. (1999). The origin of HIV–1. From Pan to pandemic. *Nature.* 397: 385–6.

CHAPTER 11 THE POTENTIAL FOR THE CONTROL OF NON-COMMUNICABLE DISEASES BY VACCINATION OR IMMUNOTHERAPY

Autoimmunity

Clark, I.A., Al-Yaman, F.M., Cowden, W.B., Rockett, K.A. (1996). Does malarial tolerance, through nitric oxide, explain the low incidence of autoimmune disease in tropical Africa? *Lancet.* 348: 1492–4.

Elliman, D. (1999). Vaccination and type 1 diabetes mellitus, *Br. Med. J.* 316: 1159–60.

Feldmann, M., Brennan, F.M., Maini, R.N. (1996). Role of cytokines in rheumatoid arthritis. *Annual Review of Immunology.* 14: 397–440.

Garcia, G. and Weiner, H.L. (1998). Manipulation of Th responses by oral tolerance. *Annual Review of Immunology.* 16: 123–146.

Pearson, C.J. and McDevitt, H.O. (1998). Redirecting Th1 and Th2 responses in autoimmune disease. In: *Redirection of Th1 and Th2 Responses.* eds R. L. Coffman and S. Romagnani. Springer, Berlin: 79–122.

Rockett, K.A., Awburn, M., Rockett, E.J., Cowden, W.B., Clark, I.A. (1994). Possible role of nitric oxide in malarial immunosuppression. Parasite Immunol. 16: 243–9.

Tian, J., Olcott, A., Hannsen, L., et al. (1999). Antigen-based immune therapy for autoimmune disease: from animal models to humans. *Immunol. Today.* 20: 190–5.

Willenborg, D.O., Fordham, S., Bernard, C., Cowden, W.B., Ramshaw, I.A. (1996). IFN-γ plays a critical down-regulatory role in the induction and effector phase of myelin oligodendrocyte glycoprotein-induced autoimmune encephalomyelitis. *J. Immunol.* 157: 3223–7.

Willenborg, D.O. and Staykova, M.A. (1998). Approaches to the treatment of central nervous system autoimmune disease using specific neuroantigen. *Immunol. Cell Biol.* 76: 91–103.

Cancer

Boon, T. and Old, L.J. (1997). Cancer tumour antigens. *Curr. Opinion in Immunology.* 9: 681–3.

Chang, M-H., Chen, C-J., Lai, M-S., et al. (1997). Universal hepatitis B vaccination in Taiwan and the incidence of hepatocellular carcinoma in children. *N. Engl. J. Med.* 336: 1855–9.

Fernando, G.J.P., Murray, B., Zhou, J., Frazer, I.H. (1999). Expression, purification and immunological characterisation of the transforming protein E7, from cervical cancer-associated human papilloma virus type 16. *Clin. Exp. Immunol.* 115: 397–403.

Finke, J., Ferron, S., Frey, A., et al. (1999). Where have all the T cells gone? Mechanisms of immune evasion by tumors. *Immunol. Today.* 20: 158–60.

Folkman, J. (1998). Antiangiogenic gene therapy. *Proc. Natl. Acad. Sci.* 95: 9064–6.

French, R.R., et al. (1999) CD40 antibody evokes a cytotoxic T-cell response that eradicates lymphoma and by-passes T-cell help. *Nature Med.* 5: 548–52.

Mahoney, F.J. and Kane, M. (1999). Hepatitis B vaccine. In: *Vaccines.* (3rd edn) eds S.A. Plotkin and W.A. Orenstein. W.B. Saunders & Co., Philadelphia: 158–182.

Nestle, F.O. and 7 others. (1998). Vaccination of melanoma patients with peptide- or tumour lysate-pulsed dendritic cells. *Nature Med.* 4: 328–32.

Ockert D., Schmitz, M., Hampl, M., Rieber, E.P. (1999). Advances in cancer immunotherapy. *Immun. Today.* 20: 63–5.

Pardoll, D. (1997). Meeting report. Maturation of cancer vaccines. *Biochem. Biophys. Acta.* 1332: R33–6.

Rosenberg, S.A. and 15 others. (1998). Immunologic and therapeutic evaluation of a synthetic peptide vaccine for the treatment of patients with metastatic melanoma. *Nature Med.* 4: 321–7.

Timmerman, J.M. and Levy, R. (1998). Melanoma vaccines: prim and proper presentation. *Nature Med.* 4: 269–70.

Timmerman, J.M. and Levy, R. (1999). Dendritic cell vaccines for cancer immunotherapy. *Ann. Rev. Medicine.* 60: 507–530.

Tulpule, A., Gill, P.S., Levine, A.M. (1998). Neoplastic complications of

HIV infection. In: *AIDS and other manifestations of HIV infection.* ed. G.P. Wormser, Lippincott-Raven, Philadelphia: 529–40.

Williams, N. 1996. Tumour cells fight back to beat immune system. *Science.* 274: 1302.

Zorn, E. and Hercend, T. (1999). A MAGE-encoded peptide is recognised by expanded lymphocytes infiltrating a spontaneously regressing human primary melanoma lesion. *Eur. J. Immunol.* 29: 602–7, and 592–601.

Fertility control

Cooperative Research Centre for Biological Control of Vertebrate Pest Populations (1998). *Annual Report.* CSIRO, Canberra, Australia.

Talwar, G.P., Singh, O., Pal, R., et al. (1994). A vaccine that prevents pregnancy in women. *Proc. Natl. Acad. Sci.* 91: 8532–6.

Talwar, G.P. and Raghupathy, R. (eds) (1995). *Birth Control Vaccines.* Medical Intelligence Unit, R.G. Landes, Austin, Tx.: 1–171.

Index
Names

Index
Topics

GERM WARFARE

Breakthroughs in immunology

ALAN G. BAXTER

'I met many of these people, count some as good friends, lived through a few of the ups and downs and was bitten by more than one genetically-defined mouse. I am also a character in this "Pilgrim's Progress" of a modern, dynamic scientific discipline. I hope that you will enjoy this "warts and all" account of a medically important and fascinating area of human enquiry.

Peter C. Doherty, Nobel Prize Winner, 1996

Whether we like it or not, our bodies play host to a horde of microscopic organisms including viruses, bacteria and worms—some of which happily co-exist with us and others which would do the dirty on us if they could. Our only defence against these potentially harmful, uninvited guests is our immune system.

Germ Warfare describes the successes of this defence system but along with the victories it also describes breaches in the defences, leading to infections and autoimmune diseases such as arthritis and multiple sclerosis. By telling the stories of the major players in this new science of immunology, Alan Baxter explodes the myth of scientists as being stooped, stammering savants and brings their colourful characters alive. The temperamental rages of Elie Metchnikoff; the gentle New England dedication of George Snell; Howard Florey, the 'Australian bushranger'; Macfarlane Burnet, deeply shy yet politically adept; and the sophisticated charm of Peter Medawar all contribute to this refreshingly honest and humorous history of the great achievers and achievements in the once secret science that affects each and every one of us.

Alan G. Baxter is the Head of the Autoimmunity Group at the Centenary Institute in Sydney. He is fortunate enough to know and have studied under some of the characters in his book.

SCIENCE

ISBN 1-86508-070-5

UNRAVELLING GENES

A layperson's guide to genetic engineering

MARK WALKER and DAVID McKAY

You don't need to be a professor of biology—or any type of scientist at all—to understand the basics of 'genetic engineering', 'cloning' and 'gene therapy'. All you need is this book.

Unravelling Genes explains the principles of genetic engineering using a minimum of jargon. You'll learn how 'genetically modified' foods are created and will understand the new technologies that led to the cloning of Dolly the sheep. Gene therapy and its application in the treatment of diseases such as Alzheimers, cystic fibrosis and haemophilia is also demystified, giving you the information you need to form your own conclusions about these cutting-edge technologies.

'This is an outstanding book, long overdue. It presents a simple and enjoyable Cook's tour of genetic engineering, which is easily understood and yet does not lose any of the sense of sophistication and excitement of this new science'.

John Mattick is Professor of Molecular Biology at the University of Queensland and Director of the Australian Genome Research Facility.

SCIENCE

ISBN 1-86508-086-1

GUIDING THE YOUNG ATHLETE

All you need to know

DAVID JENKINS and PETER REABURN

Guiding the Young Athlete is a practical and comprehensive guide for teachers, coaches and parents which will help them to develop suitable, safe and effective training programs for the child.

There are major differences between the anatomy and physiology of adults and children involved in training for health and sport but, traditionally, parents, coaches and teachers have treated children as 'miniature adults' when devising training and exercise schedules. Unlike adults, however, children are unaware of the limitations of their bodies and are therefore particularly vulnerable to injury or exhaustion while developing poor training practices and inadequate nutritional habits.

Providing the latest information and advice on exercise and fitness for young people, the authors outline the health benefits of exercise, along with practical precautionary methods to avoid over-training and injury. They also demonstrate that it is possible and, in many cases beneficial, to develop sensible training schedules for children suffering various chronic syndromes. Sensible nutritional guidelines for the child are also included.

David Jenkins and Peter Reaburn are both parents of young, active families. Former physical education teachers, they are now university lecturers in exercise physiology and sports nutrition and the editors of *Training for Speed and Endurance*.

SPORT/HEALTH

ISBN 1-86508-218-X